MOBILIZATION

FOR THE NEUROLOGICALLY INVOLVED CHILD

ASSESSMENT

AND

APPLICATION

STRATEGIES

FOR PEDIATRIC

PTs AND OTs

Sandra Brooks-Scott, M.S., PPT, PCS

Therapy
Skill Builders™ ®

a division of
The Psychological Corporation

555 Academic Court
San Antonio, Texas 78204-2498
1-800-228-0752

Copyright © 1997 by

**Therapy
Skill Builders**™ ®
a division of
The Psychological Corporation

555 Academic Court
San Antonio, Texas 78204-2498
1-800-228-0752

The *Learning Curve Design* is a registered trademark of
The Psychological Corporation.

0761643362

12   11   10   9   8   7   6   5   4   3   A   B   C   D   E

Printed in the United States of America

To my son, Ryan, and his
recovery from Guillain Barré

Acknowledgments

To the many people who encouraged, supported, critiqued, taught, and tolerated me during the endeavor known as writing a book, I can only say, "Thank you." Those who were particularly helpful include:

Deirdre, who taught me to look at the patient, not the book.

Scotty, the little boy with spastic quadriplegia, who started all of this.

Barb, the instructor who gave me both the chance to try this with Scotty and the challenge to develop the concepts into a coherent whole.

The many, many therapists and children who participated in my courses.

My office and therapy staff, without whom I could not have finished this project.

Tom, whose encouragement in editing and the publishing process kept me focused and sane.

Dad, who saw me through the tough times.

Michael, my husband, who is teaching me to stop and smell the roses.

Contents

Tables

Figures

Introduction

Purpose

This book posits two ideas, that proper joint mobilization can improve mobility in children with neurological dysfunction and that proper assessment of each system's contributions to mobility is the only way to maximize motor function. These two ideas are a reassessment of the traditional focus on the neural cause of the motor dysfunction in cerebral palsy. No longer can we assume that the pathology directly produces the motor deficit; rather it is the subsequent immobility that causes as much if not more damage than the original insult. Because immobility affects every system necessary to produce movement, the contribution of strength, flexibility, endurance, and range of motion to skill production must be assessed and treated. Realizing this increases available treatment options.

Because of minimal published research documenting age-appropriate strength, range of motion, and patterns of skill for the pediatric population, there are gaps in the data. This manual presents a framework from which the clinician can organize questions and data regarding the assessment and treatment of motor problems in children.

Consider this effort one more step in a journey of a thousand miles.

Content Overview

Chapter 1 describes the original neurological damage and the effects of the resultant immobility and chapter 2 focuses on the basic principles of mobilization. In chapter 3 the skeletal, ligamentous, and muscular anatomy of each joint is reviewed and an assessment strategy is presented for ruling out each system's contribution to abnormal movement. Chapters 4 to 10 discuss each joint's contributions to movement and describe assessment and mobilization techniques. In chapter 11 the concepts of mobilization are applied to motor skill development.

Chapter 1
Pathology and Resultant Immobility

Mobility is a worthy goal. However, before it can be achieved in a child with neurological dysfunction, certain prerequisites must be in place: normal bony alignment; normal muscle strength, flexibility and endurance; a coordinating nervous system; an efficient cardiorespiratory system; and normal connective tissue flexibility. Immobility after initial neurological insult affects all these systems, making assessment and treatment of all systems interfering with efficient mobility a paramount goal of the therapist.

Neurological Damage—Original Insult

The motor result of the neurological insult is dependent upon the age, the location, and the extent of the insult (Brann 1988; Costello et al. 1988; Nelson 1988; Pape and Wigglesworth 1979). The most widely discussed reason for brain damage in the pre-, peri- or initial postnatal stages is a change in blood pressure, causing the vessels in the developing organ to hemorrhage or become ischemic (Pape and Wigglesworth 1979). Nelson (1988) notes that most infants who live through severe asphyxia at birth do not develop cerebral palsy or mental retardation. Brann (1988), in his discussion of the effects of acute total and prolonged partial asphyxia, clearly demonstrates that the neurological changes and motor outcomes vary depending on the acuteness, duration, and severity of the asphyxia.

Because a child will not have autoregulatory mechanisms to control blood pressure until 3 months of age, excessive heat loss, abnormal partial pressures of oxygen and carbon dioxide, or fluid imbalances can affect a newborn's blood pressure, producing ischemic hypoxia and neural damage. Hypoxia is a decrease in oxygen to the nerve cell, which can occur as a result of a hemorrhage or ischemic attack. Hemorrhage occurs when blood leaves the vascular system, drowning the nerve cells, and ischemia is a decrease in blood flow to the nerves. Either event decreases the oxygen available to the nerve cell, resulting in its death.

Regardless of the proximate cause, too much or too little blood will damage the surrounding area of the brain. The areas of the brain most susceptible to damage are those that are metabolically most active (i.e., areas developing most actively at the time of insult, such as the arterial border and end zones). Ischemia or hemorrhage in the newborn of 32 weeks or less gestation most likely will damage the periventricular areas of the internal capsule, where the vascular supply is active in the maturing brain (Pape and Wigglesworth 1979). These areas usually carry fibers projecting to the lower extremities and trunk. Damage to this area frequently results in spastic diplegic cerebral palsy. By 40 weeks gestation, the most actively developing area of the brain is the cortex (Pape and Wigglesworth 1979). Localized damage here is more likely to result in quadriplegia or hemiplegia bilaterally.

Volpe (1988) discusses five types of pathology seen after an ischemic-hypoxic injury. They include selective neuronal necrosis, status marmoratus of basal ganglia and thalamus, parasagittal cerebral injury, periventricular leukomalacia, and focal or multifocal ischemic brain necrosis. The type of injury is heavily dependent upon the state of maturation of the synapses, receptors, and vascular supply. Parasagittal injury is the primary lesion of the term infant, for example, but periventricular leukomalacia is the principal ischemic lesion of the preterm infant.

The system's developmental stage at the time of insult also determines the extent of damage. During neural development, the normal process of cell multiplication generates excess neurons with more connections in both normal and abnormal locations (Kandel and Schwartz 1984). Functional pathways are used, reinforced, and maintained; interfering or less efficient pathways go unused, become malnourished, and eventually die.

If the damage occurs while excess neurons exist, the excess neurons have a possibility of being maintained and reinforced. Unusual connections, functional or not, will be the norm for that infant (Kandel and Schwartz 1984). If damage occurs after neuronal projections are established, those early, inefficient projections have already been destroyed. This damage not only produces a direct motor deficit but also reduces the coordinating input those projections send to other parts of the nervous system. Abnormalities of coordination, timing, reaction speed, and rapid alternating movements may be results of the absence of these coordinating projections.

Motor results of the neurological pathology can take many forms: ataxia, athetosis, rigidity, flaccidity, or spasticity. Some of these symptoms are associated with particular lesions. In some cases, such as ataxia and athetosis, causes of the neurological pathology have been identified and the incidence of the pathology has decreased.

Ataxia results when there is damage to the cerebellum. It was most commonly associated with the use of oxygen masks strapped around the baby's head. The strap created pressure on the soft skull damaging the underlying brain. Athetosis is more commonly associated with deposits of bilirubin in the basal ganglia, not blood pressure dyscrasias. Aggressive management of hyperbilirubinemia has decreased the incidence of athetosis. Rigidity is associated with damage to the basal ganglia. It is more frequently seen in severe brain trauma or meningitis than in hypoxic events. Flaccidity may be a result of damage to the cerebellum or peripheral nerves and can be maintained or later overshadowed by spasticity; it should not be confused with muscle weakness. Flaccidity is a decrease in stiffness; conversely, muscle weakness is an inability to create tension sufficient to raise the body part against gravity and age-appropriate resistance. Spasticity is increased stiffness clinically identified as an increased resistance to high velocity muscle stretch. It is a result of neurological damage. Similar stiffness may be mimicked by muscle spasm, emotional state, and connective tissue tightness.

Taken together, the above factors all affect stiffness. Stiffness is a set of behaviors including muscle activation, response to stretch, kinematic patterns, conscious control, fiber patterns, and passive elastic properties of muscles and ligaments (Guiliani 1991). Neurological damage does not cause stiffness, yet stiffness can be affected by it. All factors contributing to stiffness must be ruled out before spasticity is implicated as the cause of the motor problem. Consequently, before movement anomalies can be linked to manifestations of spasticity, the role of the other systems' contributions to stiffness, including spasm, weakness, and connective tissue tightness, must be ruled out. Spasm, weakness, and connective tissue tightness are often sequelae of immobility frequently seen in infants and children with neurological damage.

Immobility and its Effects

Immobility is frequently more detrimental than the damage that causes the immobility in the first place, and it affects all tissues of the body (Kessler and Hertling 1983; Kottke 1966; Salter 1978). Within days of immobility, several physiological changes occur:

➤ bones lose density

➤ muscles atrophy and weaken

➤ synapses deteriorate

➤ cardiorespiratory inefficiency develops

➤ connective tissue tightens

Bones Lose Density

Immobility results in calcium loss in bone (Cornwall 1984). Abnormal stresses on weak bones from incorrect joint alignment may be responsible for some of the malformations frequently seen in children with cerebral palsy, such as foot deformities and hip dislocations (Bleck 1987; Cusick 1990). Immobility results in permanent deformity by maintaining infantile bone shape or allowing bones to twist as in some foot deformities or scoliosis (Badgley 1949; Beals 1969; Raney and Brashear 1971; Salter 1978).

Muscles Atrophy and Weaken

The neurological damage in spastic cerebral palsy, regardless of cause or age at time of damage, decreases the correct neural input to the muscles. Abnormal neural input to the muscles in infancy has the following sequelae:

1. changes in muscle fiber differentiation and development
2. atrophy and weakness

Neural input is critical for muscle development (Kandel and Schwartz 1984). The type of neural input influences the histochemical and contractile properties of muscle fibers. These histochemical and contractile properties determine the type of muscle fiber. The type of muscle fiber determines the type of contraction the infant can create. At birth, the infant's fast and slow muscle fibers are approximately equal (Slaten 1981; Spieholz 1982). Whereas the general proportion of fast to slow fibers for each muscle is thought to be genetically predetermined, evidence exists that muscle fibers are also responsive to exercise (Astrand and Rodahl 1977; Basmajian 1975; Rose and Rothstein 1982). Normally, the infant exercises or trains muscles tonically and phasically through the full range of motion. Children with cerebral palsy train their muscles abnormally—usually tonically in only one part of the range of motion. With abnormal neural input to muscles, muscles are unable to create appropriate force, and generalized weakness follows. To perform any movement, infants with neurological damage must recruit more muscles to create the tension necessary to move. This is a normal response to the abnormal situation of weakness. The synergistic actions (often tonic) may reinforce an abnormal differentiation of the muscles. The more children with neurological damage try to move, the more they recruit. The more they recruit, the more they influence muscles to develop slow-fiber-type characteristics, which results in decreased muscle use for efficient phasic activities such as gait, balance, reach, and grasp. Therapeutic exercise must take into account the type of contraction necessary for normal movement.

The second effect of abnormal input of the nervous system on muscles is atrophy and weakness. Immobility causes atrophy, but the effects of immobility on muscle fiber types differ depending on the cause of immobility. According to Rose and Rothstein (1982), there is a preferential atrophy of slow-twitch fibers in cast immobility, but mixed atrophy occurs in osteoarthritis. Because children with cerebral palsy are generally less mobile than their peers, frequently casted (preferential slow fiber atrophy), and often develop osteoarthritis (mixed atrophy), it is reasonable to assess the strength of the child's muscle for both slow- and fast-twitch activities. Patients with neurological deficits show a change, sometimes even a reversal, in the normal fiber proportion in many muscles (Rosenflack and Andreasson 1980; Saltin and Landen 1975). For example, the gastrocsoleous is a predominantly fast-twitch muscle used phasically in gait, yet many clients with neurological damage show an increase in slow-twitch fibers. Consequently, the increased slow-twitch fiber proportion may interfere with the phasic activity of push-off in gait. Specific phasic exercises would be necessary to address this problem. Therapeutic activities can then be designed to address strength for both fast- and slow-twitch activities.

Beyond assessing overall strength, it is essential to identify where in the range of motion the strength occurs. Research on patients with neurological damage (Gate et al. 1986; Kramer and MacPhail 1994; Vaughan 1989) suggests that patients have isometric strength in some parts of the range of motion, but not isokinetic strength throughout the range of motion. Because isometric strength tends to be in the range the patient uses (quadriceps strength at 20-degree knee flexion in the child with spastic diplegic cerebral palsy), training in specific ranges and type of contraction may improve the expression of motor function.

Neurological Changes Occur

It has been well documented that direct damage to the brain not only destroys the damaged neuron but also the cells to which the damaged neuron connects (Kandel and Schwarz 1985). This transneuronal degeneration can affect not only neurons in synaptic contact with the damaged cell but also their peripheral target, such as muscles. For example, decreased neural input to the muscle changes the concentration of synaptic receptors at the end plate. Decreased muscle activity subsequent to decreased neural input decreases the concentration of receptors at the muscle end plate while increasing the concentration of synaptic receptors in the extrajunctional region. Consequently, the initial brain damage can cause degeneration in nondamaged neurons and muscles. Subsequent immobility decreases the input back to the nervous system.

Cardiorespiratory Inefficiency Develops

Many children with neurological damage also have lung damage, such as a thickening in the membrane walls (Hyaline Membrane Disease) or damaged alveolar walls (emphysema), resulting in decreased surface area for gas exchange. Either way, there is a physiological decrease in the ability to adjust gas exchange as metabolic demands increase with increased movement.

Under normal movement conditions, infants and children automatically challenge the cardiorespiratory system during play to develop adequate endurance for most activities. Children with cerebral palsy often lack adequate endurance for even simple motor tasks (Astrand and Rodahl 1977). Not even considering poor initial endurance, children with cerebral palsy also usually expend more energy performing tasks than children without cerebral palsy (Kramer and MacPhail 1994). This is clearly demonstrated in gait studies comparing ambulation with and without assistance devices (Astrand and Rodahl 1977; Kramer and MacPhail 1994). Pediatric therapy programs must assess and address this issue for improved motor performance to carry over from a therapeutic setting to functional activities.

Many children with cerebral palsy are limited by both cardiorespiratory and muscular deconditioning. For the child with muscular deconditioning, the exercise of choice must also train the specific muscle for the specific type of work desired. Swimming can provide excellent training for a child's quadriceps, but may do little to train the gastrocsoleous for the phasic contractions against body weight necessary in walking. Implications for treatment include cardiorespiratory output and exercise design.

Cardiorespiratory Output

Because muscles require oxygen and the removal of carbon dioxide to perform, the greater the muscular work required, the more efficient the gas exchange must be. As muscular effort increases, so does respiratory and cardiac output. Initially during exercise, there is an increased need for oxygen in the tissues until a steady state is achieved. There is a gradual increase in the normal child's ability to take oxygen as the lungs mature. For example, maximum oxygen uptake in a 5-year-old is 1 liter/minute, but maximum oxygen uptake in a 20-year-old rises to 3.8 liters/minute (Giannestras 1973). Respiratory frequency declines as a child grows because of the increased lung size, decreased airway resistance, and increased compliance.

The cardiac output (heart rate **x** stroke volume) increases as muscular work increases, providing oxygen to and removing carbon dioxide from the muscles. Increased cardiac output results from an increase in stroke volume, not increased heart rate. Maximal heart rate changes only slightly with age: Mean resting heart rate for children 4 to 12 years old (with and without cerebral palsy) was 100 beats per minute. Ambulation in children with and without cerebral palsy raised the average heart rate to 160 beats per minute (Astrand and Rodahl 1977).

Both hypoactivity and the muscle weakness from the neurological condition in cerebral palsy decrease the child's overall conditioning. Additional factors (e.g., heart conditions and chronic respiratory conditions) contribute to the deconditioning. The high mechanical inefficiency of motion in children with cerebral palsy contributes to the high metabolic cost of even simple tasks, not to mention activities of daily living.

Exercise Design

Four factors to consider in designing an exercise program to improve cardiorespiratory endurance include type, intensity, frequency, and duration of exercise. Type of exercise should consider flexibility, strength, and each child's interest as well as the availability of necessary equipment. High intensity anaerobic exercise such as sprinting and weightlifting will not provide the cardiorespiratory endurance effects necessary in the child but may provide isolated strength training (Bar-Or 1983). Low-impact rhythmic activities—such as walking or propelling a wheelchair, swimming, dancing, horseback riding, and basketball—are more likely to improve cardiorespiratory endurance.

Intensity of training must be child-specific and based upon oxygen uptake or heart rate. Although oxygen uptake is not easily measured in the clinic, heart rate is. For healthy individuals, training occurs at 60 to 90 percent of the individual's maximum heart rate, perhaps too high for the deconditioned child. Giannestras (1973) recommends a 50 to 65 percent rate, which may be better suited for this population. The suggestion of the "talk test" is also a reasonable way to monitor the child's exercise tolerance. The "talk test" encourages the child to start exercising slowly but increase the intensity until breathing is moderately increased while speaking (i.e., talking is somewhat labored).

Benefits of training have been documented when frequency of training occurs between two and four times per week. Note, however, that this does not mean children must participate in therapy that often. If the exercise is something children enjoy, they can perform it and benefit without the therapist's presence. During therapy, therapists can monitor change and increase a program's difficulty as appropriate. Skills sometimes improve when therapy becomes less frequent, but only when the caregiver associates those skills with daily functional activities understood by the children (Bower and McClellan 1992).

Duration of the training is dependent upon the individual child's attention span and ability to perform the task. The heart rate, however, must be maintained for 15 to 30 minutes for any training to take effect. Therapy sessions with frequent gaps seldom build cardiorespiratory or muscular endurance. Giannestras (1973) recommends beginning with training periods of 10 to 15 minutes and working up to 30 to 40 minutes. Walking to a friend's house, the playground, or around the mall can not only be excellent training activities, but are also frequently age-appropriate, functional, and a whole lot more fun than "therapy."

Connective Tissue Tightens

Immobility also changes connective tissue. Prenatal immobility may interfere in normal joint development, resulting in congenital contractures (Davis and Kalousek 1988; Viljoen et al. 1989). Postnatally, contractures are caused by the reorganization of the connective tissue fibers (Threlkeld 1992).

Postnatally, simple immobility affects ligaments, resulting in a net loss of mucopolysaccharide content, but collagen content remains constant. The loss of lubricant may enable collagen fibers to approximate and form abnormal cross-links that inhibit the fiber's ability to glide, reducing tissue extensibility (Threlkeld 1992). Any limitation of the joint connective tissue will mimic an inflexible or short muscle. Consequently, joint limitation must be ruled out prior to concluding that abnormal range of motion is due to a short muscle.

Threlkeld (1992) observed that connective tissue structures, especially fiber orientation and cross links, are strongly dependent upon the applied loads. However, children with cerebral palsy cannot apply those loads or forces across the cartilage independently or in a "normal" manner. Consequently, the child with cerebral palsy has difficulty reducing the normal prenatal contractures (such as at the hip) and preventing new ones from forming due to relatively static postures (such as at the ankle).

Even if pain is absent, joint pathology can inhibit muscle activity, leading to weakness and wasting (Stokes and Young 1984). This may be part of the vicious cycle of immobility seen in children with cerebral palsy: The child is born with brain damage, which limits the creation of muscle force; this limits movement against gravity, which creates changes in the joint, bone, muscle, nerve, cardiac, and respiratory tissues; this leads to more difficulty in generating muscle force, which in turn limits movement. An assessment of motor performance addressing all systems contributing to poor skill performance provides an expanded treatment repertoire to improve efficiency of motor performance in children with cerebral palsy.

Treatment Implications

By expanding the concept of "brain damage leads to spasticity, which leads to poverty of movement" to "brain damage leads to immobility, which leads to physiological effects on the tissues, which leads to poverty of movement" more treatment options become available. This change in concept expands the possible causes of the motor deficits seen in patients as well as the treatment options to address those deficits.

For example, in the first model, sacral-sitting can be viewed as a result of increased tone with a treatment option to decrease tone. Under the proposed model, however, sacral-sitting may be due to increased tone, limited hip joint connective tissue flexibility, weak hamstrings, short hamstrings, or any combination. Decreasing tone will only address one possible factor with no effect on other factors contributing to the sacral sitting. Mobilization may be necessary for hip joint periarticular connective tissue flexibility of 90 to 120 degrees. Stretching the hamstrings may be necessary to achieve muscle flexibility in the 120 degree range of hip flexion. Strengthening the hamstrings eccentrically from 90 to 120 degrees of hip flexion may be necessary to control the sway of body weight forward in sitting. Treatment must be directed to the cause of that individual's reason for sacral-sitting. Specific assessment that rules out competing explanations for the motor symptom in the given individual focuses treatment to the specific cause of the motor symptom in that individual. Many resources address the contribution of tone to poor motor performance. This manual focuses on the contribution of periarticular and muscular causes of poor motor performance.

Summary

There are many types of pathology affecting the nervous system, resulting in the movement disorders in cerebral palsy. The neural pathology not only directly produces motor deficits, but also causes relative immobility. This relative immobility indirectly produces motor deficits because of its effects on the skeleton, muscles, nerves, heart, lungs, and ligaments. The contribution of these indirect motor deficits to the child's motor performance must be assessed and treated before assuming the performance exhibited by the child is due to the original neural insult.

Chapter 2
Principles of Mobilization

In the literature on the management of children with cerebral palsy, the focus has been on neurological approaches. No texts have discussed application of mobilization to the management of cerebral palsy. Before mobilization can be applied to the management of cerebral palsy, an overview of mobilization is necessary.

This chapter discusses techniques designed to stretch extra-articular structures of synovial joints. Key concepts to consider in the application of the techniques are joint play, grades of motion, close-packed or open-packed positions, and the rule of convex and concave.

Joint Play

Joint play is the term for the accessory movements that can be passively but not actively performed at the joint (Kessler and Hertling 1983; Maitland 1977) and that enable smooth gliding of joint surfaces. Joint play is achieved when the extra-articular connective tissue structures are flexible enough to allow normal roll and spin of the articular surfaces, a prerequisite for normal active range of motion. To achieve normal joint play, grades of motion are applied in open-pack positions in the direction determined by the rule of convex and concave.

Grades of Motion

Grades of motion are the passive rhythmic oscillations applied to a joint to increase its extra-articular connective tissue flexibility (Kessler and Hertling 1983; Maitland 1977). Choice of grade to use depends on the joint's irritability and degree of restriction. Four grades of motion are defined (see Figure 2.1). Grades 1 and 2 decrease irritability in inflamed or painful joints, and Grades 3 and 4 increase flexibility in joints with extra-articular joint restrictions. Grades 3 and 4 are frequently used in patients with neurological impairment to increase the flexibility of joint structures that have tightened after immobility. Because these joints are seldom in acute trauma, grades 1 and 2 are used less frequently.

Close-Pack/Open-Pack Positions

In a joint's close-packed position, joint surfaces are maximally congruent; also, capsule and ligaments become twisted, causing the joint surfaces to approximate and lock so maximum stability is achieved (Kessler and Hertling 1983; Maitland 1977). Any other position is open-pack for that joint.

Table 2.1 lists the major joints and their close-packed positions. Notice that all the close-packed positions are positions in which the joint has a stability function (i.e., single limb stance is close-packed).

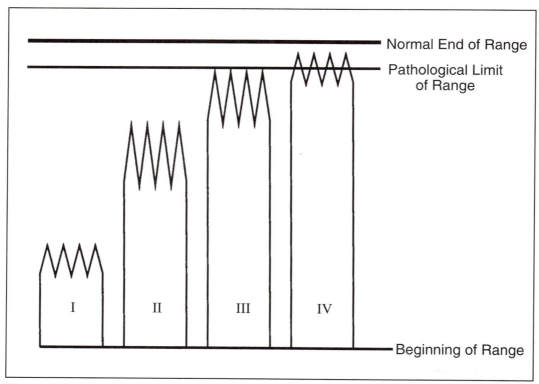

Figure 2.1. Grades of Motion
Reproduced by permission of The Saunders Group, Inc. © 1996

Table 2.1
Close-Pack Positions for the Joints

Joint	Close-Pack Position
Hip	Full extension with adduction, and internal rotation.
Knee	Full extension with external rotation.
Ankle	Full dorsiflexion for talocrural joint; supination for subtalor and midtarsal joints.
Shoulder	Maximal abduction and external rotation.
Elbow	Full extension/supination for humeroulnar joint; elbow flexion at 90° and supination at 5° for humeroradial joint.
Wrist	Full extension with radial deviation.

Rule of Convex and Concave

The rule of convex and concave determines the direction in which force is applied to achieve a desired range. Articular surfaces move relative to the shafts depending upon whether the convex or concave surface is stabilized or fixed. Hence, if the concave surface is stabilized (as the tibia in non-weightbearing dorsiflexion), the convex articular surface of the talus moves in the opposite direction of the shaft (body) of the talus. Conversely, if the convex talus is fixed (as in standing), the concave surface of the tibia moves in the same direction as the shaft of the tibia to achieve dorsiflexion. Figure 2.2 illustrates this concept. Applying this rule, the head of the talus must glide posteriorly relative to the tibia to achieve ankle dorsiflexion.

Table 2.2 summarizes the major movements used in mobilization for the neurologically impaired client.

Table 2.2
Common Mobilization Techniques for the Neurologically Impaired Child

Desired Motion	Direction of Force
Hip flexion	Femur glides posteriorly and inferiorly.
Hip extension	Femur glides anteriorly.
Hip abduction	Femur glides medially and inferiorly.
Knee extension	If in the last 15° of extension, tibia glides externally; if greater than the last 15° of extension, tibia glides anteriorly.
Knee flexion	If in the last 15° of extension, tibia glides internally; if greater than the last 15° on extension, the tibia glides posteriorly.
Ankle dorsiflexion	Talus glides posteriorly and the fibula and tibia separate at the mortise.
Shoulder flexion	Humerus glides inferiorly, clavicle depresses and rotates at the sternal articulation.
Shoulder abduction	Humerus glides inferiorly, clavicle depresses and rotates at the sternal articulation.
Supination	Head of the radius rotates on the ulna.
Wrist extension	Capitate glides palmarly on the scaphoid, the scaphoid glides dorsally on the lunate, then the scaphoid glides palmarly on the radius.

General Rules of Mobilization

The following are five general rules to observe while using mobilization techniques:

1. The patient must be relaxed.
2. The therapist must be relaxed.
3. One hand stabilizes a body part while the other hand mobilizes its articulating part.
4. The therapist considers the direction of movement, the velocity of movement, and the amplitude of movement.
5. One movement at a time, one joint at a time.

Indications and Contraindications

Joint mobilization is indicated when the extra-articular connective tissue abnormally restricts motion of that joint. For example, babies have a 60-degree hip flexion contracture at birth due to connective tissue tightness (Lee 1977). Many children with cerebral palsy also have a hip flexion contracture due to connective tissue tightness. Mobilization of the hip joint in infants is contraindicated because they have normal limitations and the ability to overcome them with their own oscillatory end-range movements when kicking. Mobilization would be indicated in the older child with cerebral palsy exhibiting abnormal range limitations interfering with function caused by extra-articular tissue tightness.

Contraindications fall into four categories:

1. Risk of fracture. The forces in mobilization can cause fractures in weak bones. Osteogenesis imperfecta or a history of pathological fractures is a contraindication to mobilization.

2. Joint inflammation. Stretching of articular tissue is contraindicated when the tissue itself is under stress such as the stretch from inflammation, as in acute juvenile rheumatoid arthritis.

3. Desired hypomobility. Extra-articular tissue stretching is contraindicated when fixation is required. Mobilization would be contraindicated at the subtalor joint following a triple arthrodesis in a child with cerebral palsy but may be indicated at the talocrural joint subsequent to the immobility from the casting for the surgery.

4. Hypermobility. Excessive mobility in a given direction at a specific joint is a contraindication to mobilization, but the techniques may be appropriate in a different direction at the same joint or in a related joint. For example, it is contraindicated to mobilize the glenohumeral joint in a child with cerebral palsy with a tendency to sublux the glenohumeral joint, but mobilization of the sternoclavicular joint may be indicated to increase shoulder girdle range of motion without stressing the glenohumeral joint.

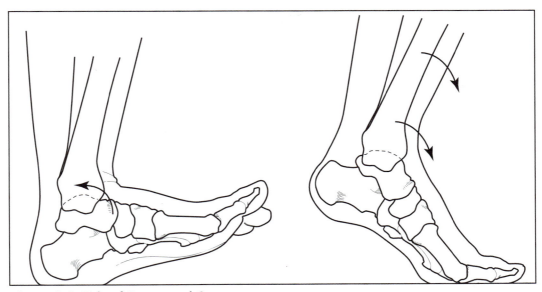

Figure 2.2. Rule of Convex and Concave

Effectiveness of Mobilization

Little evidence exists for effectiveness of mobilization in adults with orthopedic problems, but some evidence does exist for effectiveness of mobilization to improve range of motion in children with neurological problems.

Hoesli (1988) used a single-subject design to assess the effects of hip joint inferior glide mobilization techniques on a 7-year-old child with cerebral palsy. Initial range of motion measurements were taken after the regular therapeutic regimen. Subsequently, mobilization was added to the regimen and measured after four weeks of treatment for a total of 11 measurements. Hoesli found a 26-degree improvement in hip flexion at the left hip and 29-degree improvement in hip flexion at the right hip. More important, that increased range provided enough mobility at the hip joint to shift the center of gravity forward over the base of support for better sitting balance.

Brooks (1990) reports the results of the inferior glide technique on the sitting posture in 10 children who sacral-sit. The 10 randomly selected children agreed to participate in a demonstration of the mobilization technique during postgraduate courses presented over a 3-year period. All of the children would sacral-sit in tailor- or ring-sitting (i.e., they sat with a rounded spine with weight on the sacrum). Maximum hip flexion was measured at less than 90 degrees in all 10 children. An inferior glide technique was used to increase hip flexion greater than 90 degrees. Increases in range of hip flexion averaged 25 degrees and resulted in placement of the center of gravity over the base of support for better sitting balance. The children were able to place the weight over the legs in tailor-sitting. A similar strategy was reported in Brooks (1994) on a child treated by a participant in one of the courses.

Mobilization does not affect spasticity, but may affect muscle spasms, the connective tissue component of stiffness, and the range of motion necessary to

➤ place the center of gravity over the base of support for improved function,

➤ gain strength in a position of improved efficiency for muscle function, and

➤ practice the rapid alternating movements between opposing muscles necessary for balance.

Harris and Lundgren (1991) raise the concern regarding use of a technique that has not been well researched as to its effectiveness or side effects. It is critical to document the effectiveness of intervention strategies, to collect accurate data, to interpret the data carefully, and to assess and implement strategies effectively. This manual presents an assessment approach that analyzes movement by each joint. Many children with cerebral palsy present clinically similar movement patterns, but assessment frequently reveals different causes for the motor performance. Different causes of the movement dysfunction require different treatment approaches for successful and efficient intervention.

Summary

Joint play is the accessory motion that can be passively but not actively performed at a joint. To achieve normal joint play when there is a restriction secondary to periarticular connective tissue tightness, the therapist must consider grades of motion applied in an open-packed position in the direction dictated by the rule of convex and concave. Mobilization is contraindicated when there is a significant risk of fracture, joint inflammation, desired hypomobility, or joint hypermobility. Effectiveness of mobilization in adult acute orthopedic problems is controversial. However, several studies of mobilization of the hip joint in children with cerebral palsy do suggest improved range of motion resulting in correct placement of the center of gravity over the base of support in sitting. Subsequent chapters address assessment and treatment applications at each joint.

The neurological deficit in cerebral palsy results in motor dyscrasias subsequent to the neurological deficit; relative immobility frequently occurs as a result. Between the effects of the primary neurological insult and the secondary effects of immobility, all systems of the body are affected. Poor motor performance in children with neurological insults can be a result of the influence of any system. Chapter 3 outlines a system assessment designed to determine the specific cause of a given motor performance.

Chapter 3
System Assessment

The following chapters review the skeletal, ligamentous, and muscular anatomy of each joint and present an assessment strategy for sequentially ruling out each system's contribution to abnormal motion at that joint. This approach tailors specific measurable goals and treatment programs to specific deficits and differentiates children with comparable diagnoses but different causes for similar motor patterns.

This chapter proposes an assessment protocol to determine each system's contribution to the individual child's motor performance. Whereas any two children may have similar sitting or walking patterns, each child has a unique combination of range, strength, endurance, and motor-planning abilities.

Skeletal System

Bone alignment and joint range of motion must be considered in any assessment of the skeletal system. Bone alignment influences motor performance, as with femoral or tibial torsion. Joint range of motion influences the center of gravity over the base of support, as well as the total motion available regardless of strength or motor control.

Genetic and environmental factors underpin bone alignment. Very little can be done about the genetic predisposition of overall bone shape. However, the environment influences bone shape through Wolff's law (Leveau and Bernhardt 1984): Tissues grow based on stresses placed upon them—namely, gravity and muscle pull. An imbalance of or lack of muscle forces secondary to non-weightbearing may lead to skeletal deformation (Leveau and Bernhardt 1984) as in scoliosis, or a maintenance of infantile shape, as in the hip of the child with cerebral palsy. This muscle imbalance and lack of weightbearing may be responsible for the high incidence of immature and abnormally shaped bones in children with cerebral palsy.

To assess alignment, issues to consider include: a) is alignment normal for the age? and b) what forces are necessary to mold alignment as the child grows?

More frequently, range of motion is limited not by bone alignment but by connective tissue limitations. These could be ligamentous or muscular.

Ligamentous System

Limitations to range of motion from extra-articular connective tissue may be normal as in hip flexion in the newborn, or knee extension in the child. Abnormal limitations often prevent the center of gravity from moving over the base of support, interfering with efficient movement.

To assess range of motion, issues to consider include: a) is joint play available and normal for age in all directions? and b) is passive range of motion available and normal for age in all directions? Alignment and available range of motion are discussed for each joint in subsequent chapters. Many chapters contain few documented range of motion norms for children because they are lacking in the literature. Although this is a gap in the text, it can be seen as a challenge to researchers.

Reliability

Though the age-appropriate norms have not been documented, reliability of range of motion measurements in children has been reported. Numerous researchers consistently have found a 5 to 10 degree variation in interrater reliability at multiple joints in children with neurological impairment. This is an accepted variation. Consequently, a change attributed to therapeutic procedures must be greater than this 5 to 10 degree variation. Ashton et al. (1978) reported reliability coefficients ranging from $r=.33$ to $r=.82$ for hip measurements made by 16 therapists on four children with spastic diplegia. Bartlett et al. (1985) found reliability coefficients of $r=.70$ to $r=.84$ for interrater measurements of hip flexion contractures in 15 children with spastic diplegia. Rothstein et al. (1983) found a similar pattern with intrarater reliability higher ($r=.91$ to $r=.99$) than test interrater ($r=.63$ to $r=.70$) for elbows and knees in 24 patients. Ankle and foot measures were reliable for intrarater reliability ($r=.74$ to $r=.90$) according to Elveru et al. (1988), but interrater testing was not reliable. Stuberg et al. (1989) found similar patterns.

Though interrater and intrarater reliability for range of motion has been determined, it is very difficult to determine reliably which grade of motion is applied within the range of joint play. Few studies have been done to determine the reliability of joint play assessment. No studies to assess reliability of joint play assessment in children have been completed. Advances in technology may help correct the problem. In the meantime, the practice of learning from a skilled clinician is required.

Muscular System

Assessment of the muscular system involves three different variables: flexibility, strength, and endurance. Flexibility is the muscle's ability to stretch to a given length; strength, the muscle's ability to create tension; and endurance, the muscle's ability to maintain a contraction or to repeatedly contract and relax fast enough and long enough for function.

Flexibility

Muscle flexibility must be distinguished from joint flexibility. Common tests for muscle flexibility assume normal underlying joint flexibility, but this assumption must be questioned in the child with cerebral palsy. For example, the common tests of hamstring flexibility assume full hip and knee range of motion. In the straight leg raise, at least 90 degrees of hip flexion and full knee extension are required to show the frequently quoted norm of 90 degree straight leg raise. There are two problems with this test in the child with cerebral palsy. First, 80 degrees is the norm for a straight leg raise in the adult (Kendall and McCreary 1983), not 90 degrees. There is no evidence that children have more range of motion in the straight leg raise. Second, even with the hamstrings on slack, as when the knee is flexed, children with cerebral palsy seldom have 90 degrees or more hip flexion without substitution, nor do they always have full knee extension.

These difficulties interpreting hamstring flexibility still exist when the popliteal angle test is used. The popliteal angle test assumes 90 degrees of hip flexion as a starting position, then measures the knee angle as an indicator of hamstring flexibility. If the hip does not have 90 degrees of flexion and the knee does not have full extension, the test is not a measure of hamstring flexibility. Rather, it is an indicator of limited range either from one or both of the joint limitations or a combination of the joint limitation and muscle flexibility.

Because muscle flexibility testing is commonly used in the assessment of children with cerebral palsy, it is also critical to consider the rotational nature of the planes of normal joint motion when interpreting data from flexibility testing of infants and small children (Van Sant 1989). Although the cardinal planes make learning the concepts of flexibility testing easier, it is not the alignment consistent with the human body and certainly not consistent with the alignment in infants (Van Sant 1989). Consequently, someone testing the hamstring flexibility in a 3-month-old will need to consider the diagonal nature of the hip joint, whereas someone testing hamstring flexibility in an 18-year-old can follow patterns of adult testing.

Validity of muscle flexibility testing is dependent upon ruling out alternative variables that may interfere with test interpretation. Joint limitation and bone torsion are variables that must be ruled out before accurate interpretation of the results will provide effective intervention strategies.

Studies on the reliability of muscle flexibility testing suggest high variability in interrater testing. This may be due to differences in expected norms, as well as differences in environment and force so frequently seen when a child is tested at home and then again at the hospital clinic.

Strength

The second characteristic of the muscular system is strength. Strength is the ability of a muscle to create tension (Basmajian 1975), and it can be measured as the active contraction of a muscle against gravity and against resistance without substitution (Daniels and Worthingham 1972; Kendall and McCreary 1983). Isometric assessment is referred to as the break test (i.e., how much resistance can a muscle accept in a given point in the range before the muscle gives or "breaks"). In contrast, eccentric and concentric assessments are "brake" tests (i.e., how much resistance can a muscle accept in a lengthening or shortening contraction).

Strength in one kind of contraction or in one part of the range of motion does not presume strength in another kind of contraction or part of the range. This is especially true when testing children with cerebral palsy (Rosenflack and Andreasson 1980, among others). Traditionally, patients with neurological injuries are not considered weak (Bobath 1980), and one cannot measure muscle strength in the patient with a neurological injury because of the spastic synergies (Bobath 1980). Clinicians, however, routinely measure progress in their patients by the patient's increased strength with no objective reference for the term. Researchers have also suggested that patients with neurological damage do, in fact, have weakness in specific parts of their range of motion (Damiano et al. 1996; Rosenflack and Andreasson 1980; Saltin and Landen 1975). Not only is individual muscle group weakness a problem in motor control for children with neurological damage, but so is the imbalance in strength between opposing groups. This is obvious after a posterior rhizotomy (Staudt and Peacock 1989).

Strength Assessment

Considerations in accurate strength testing include isolated vs. synergistic muscle action, type of contraction, substitution, and grading.

Very few muscles work in isolation. Normal action is a combination of agonists, synergists, and antagonists. For example, hip flexors are not tested in isolation, but as a group. A muscle grade is given for the primary contraction antigravity, through the range and against an amount of resistance before significant substitution occurs.

This definition can be applied to muscle strength in the child with cerebral palsy if care is taken to stop the test at the point where the child recruits excess muscle to complete an action (i.e., substitutes). For example, a child tries to raise his or her right arm. From 0 to 30 degrees the arm flexes at the shoulder without evidence of substitution. At 30 degrees the elbow flexes, the spine flexes, and the child laterally tilts. One explanation for this is weakness of the shoulder flexors. A second explanation is synergistic action subsequent to neural damage. To determine which is the case for a given child, a strengthening exercise program is developed. Starting strength is based on observed motion. In this example, if the shoulder flexes partial range antigravity with little resistance (P+ or F-) before the child substitutes (i.e., shortens the lever arm by bending the elbow and using lateral trunk flexion to apparently raise the arm), an exercise program designed to increase strength of the shoulder flexors prior to the substitution should allow the child to increase range of motion at the shoulder while maintaining the extended elbow. If neural synergy is the cause, the strengthening program will not affect the tendency of the elbow to flex and the spine to curve when the shoulders are elevated.

The ability to contract the muscle groups necessary for function, and strength in the correct type of contraction is critical. The three types of contraction (isometric, concentric, and eccentric) require differences in the basic test procedure. For example, an isometric contraction is the ability to hold a position against gravity and resistance, and a concentric contraction requires a muscle to move a body part through the range and against both gravity and resistance. It is possible to have a good grade muscle in an isometric contraction (as the quadriceps in a standing child with spastic diplegia at 20 degrees of knee flexion), yet have only fair grade muscle in a concentric contraction (as the quadriceps in a sitting child with spastic diplegia trying to fully extend the knee). Because specific strength for a specific activity is needed, training for the necessary type of strength must consider type of contraction. Isokinetic knee extensor strength was somewhat related to walking efficiency and gross motor ability in adolescents with cerebral palsy (Kramer and MacPhail 1994). Training for as little as 8 weeks can make a difference for adults. Damiano et al. (1996) have addressed quadriceps strengthening in children with cerebral palsy, noting improved function with improved strength subsequent to quadriceps strength training.

A third consideration in strength assessment is substitution. Substitution can occur by moving another part to mimic the required action, recruiting extra muscle, or by changing the test position. It is possible that children with cerebral palsy use common substitutions (as in the example of the arm raise above), but the substitutions are viewed as synergy patterns or increased tone. Differentiating weakness (which requires increased recruitment to perform an action) from synergy patterns or increased tone directly influences the choice of treatment. Strengthening would be appropriate if weakness were present, but tone-reducing activities are more appropriate if increased resistance to passive stretch (i.e., spasticity), is determined as the cause of the poor motor performance.

The fourth consideration in assessing strength is the definition of grades. If strength were measured in terms of adult norms, all children would be relatively weak. Children simply cannot take the same amount of resistance as an adult. A 2-year-old would be weak in terms of adult norms because of an inability to lift a 20-pound bag of groceries. Similarly, a 2-year-old with cerebral palsy would be weak because of an inability to lift a 3-ounce spoon. Even though there is a significant difference in the strength between these two children, both would receive a fair grade if adult norms were used. By defining strength in terms of age-related abilities, a 2-year-old would be normal if he or she could lift and throw a ball 10 feet in a straight line (Folio and Fewel 1983). The 2-year-old with cerebral palsy may have only fair strength if able to complete the range necessary to throw the ball without substitution but could not complete the range against the resistance of the ball.

The increase in the child's ability to accept resistance can be measured by weighing the common objects children lift, kick, or otherwise manipulate. Increasing the child's ability from lifting a 3-ounce spoon to lifting a 3-ounce spoon with 3 ounces of food on it without substitution is not only a significant increase in strength (doubling), but also a significant increase in function (self-feeding). "Normal" requires full range antigravity movement against age-appropriate resistance. It is normal, therefore, for an infant to show partial-range antigravity no-resistance quadriceps activity at birth (when the knee does not usually have full extension), but that is only fair strength for the toddler kicking a ball.

There is little organized strength criteria for children. Tables in each chapter suggest clinical measures of strength in different ages based on commonly found gross and fine motor assessments (Bailey 1993; Folio and Fewel 1983). These tests were chosen because they are familiar to pediatric therapists and present skills at a given age on a normative population. There are many reasons other than strength why a child may or may not be able to do these skills. The interpretation of the data must take into account all factors in the total assessment affecting the child's movement and present a consistent explanation of the motor performance demonstrated.

Reliability of Muscle Testing

Reliability of muscle testing in children has been studied with the use of dynamometers and Cybex machines. Stuberg (1988) used a dynamometer to test intrarater and test-retest isometric muscle strength in 14 children, ages 6 to 14, with muscular dystrophy and 14 age-matched children with no muscle disease. Strength was assessed for hip and knee extension, elbow flexion, and shoulder abduction. Correlation coefficient was .83 to .99 for children with muscle disease and .74 to .99 for children without muscle disease.

Kramer and MacPhail (1994) assessed reliability of isokinetic strength testing using a Cybex to test adolescents with mild neurological involvement. They found test-retest reliability to be greater than .75 with the Cybex for this population. More involved children could not be assessed in his study because they did not have enough strength, coordination, or cognitive ability to use the equipment.

The proposed strength items have not been tested for reliability for muscle testing. They are frequently used informally in the clinic to document that children are "slightly better" after therapy or surgery because they can now perform these items. Because the items are used informally without a consistent pattern, this attempt to standardize terms and apply them clinically to children with cerebral palsy is intended to be a starting point for discussion and research. Until reliability and validity can be determined, clinical notation should define a muscle strength grade in terms of function (i.e., fair strength is the ability to move the part full range antigravity with no resistance).

Endurance

Muscular endurance can be a problem for children with neurological impairments. Children who can perform two to three repetitions of a muscle contraction but then begin to substitute other muscles may be showing poor muscular endurance. Functional mobility often requires frequent contractions. For example, if a normal child ambulates 150 steps per minute, the gastrocnemius unilaterally contracts 75 times in a minute. Now, if the child with cerebral palsy shows appropriate length and strength in the gastrocsoleous but still can only ambulate a few steps with appropriate push-off, the problem in carryover outside of therapy may be one of muscular endurance. Specific techniques to increase endurance must then be integrated into the therapeutic program to achieve functional carryover.

Neurological System

Neurological examinations assess the patient's ability to sense and process a stimulus. This information will give clues about the patient's neural damage and the particular stimuli most likely to elicit responses. A cranial nerve assessment can be critical in determining treatment options for children with cerebral palsy, because they often have multiple neuro-logical deficits. To perform a cranial nerve assessment, gather together vials of different scents to test the olfactory nerve; a pencil for visual tracking; and a piece of cotton and a safety pin for the light touch and sharp/dull discrimination. See Table 3.1 for a summary of cranial nerves, their functions, and common deficits.

Table 3.1
Cranial Nerve Assessment

Nerve	Function	Deficits
Olfactory	Sense of smell	Loss of sense of smell (with accompanying decrease in the ability to taste)
Optic	Vision	Loss of vision
Oculomotor	Movement of eyeball	Ptosis, external stabismus, dilatation of pupil, loss of power of accommodation, and slight prominence of eyeball
Trochlear	Superior oblique muscle of eyeball	Cannot turn eye downward and outward. Eye twists inward, producing double vision
Trigeminal	Mastication and sensory nerve of head and face	Face paralyzed on one or both sides; diminished salivation and lachrymal activity; paralysis of lower jaw
Abducens	Focusing element of eye	Squinting, pupil contraction
Facial	Control of facial expression	Facial paralysis or spasms
Auditory	Hearing	Unilateral or complete deafness
Glossopharyngeal	Gag reflex	Increased risk of aspiration
Vagus	Controls motor function of breathing, voice, pharynx, esophagus, stomach, and heart	Difficulty breathing, coughing, swallowing, phonating
Accessory	Motor control of trapezoids and sternocleidomastoids	Difficulty with movement in cervical spine and sternoclavicular joint
Hypoglossal	Motor control of tongue	Difficulty with speech and swallowing

Other types of nervous system assessments include proprioception; sensory discrimination (such as stereognosis and two-point discrimination); motor planning; and cerebellar functioning and critical thinking. In-depth discussion of neurological assessment can be found in many texts and will not be discussed here.

Summary

This chapter presented an assessment protocol for motor problems in children with cerebral palsy. The protocol rules out the contributions of skeletal, ligamentous, and muscular systems to motor performance before addressing the neurological contributions. A review of the literature regarding the reliability and validity of the assessment issues in children with cerebral palsy highlights considerations in interpreting assessment data. Subsequent chapters apply this protocol to movement issues on a joint-by-joint basis.

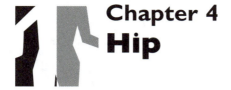

Chapter 4
Hip

Proper assessment of each system's contributions and limitations to a movement disorder is the first step toward proper mobilization. Assessing one system at a time also makes therapy both specific and efficient. Therefore, each chapter that discusses a specific joint will follow the model presented here: a section on each system, followed by a section on treatment planning or applied procedures. Addressing the hip joint first is crucial because movement of the pelvis over the femurs directly affects placement of the center of gravity over the base of support in both functional sitting and standing.

Skeletal System

The femur articulates with the three bones of the pelvis (the ilium, the pubis, and the ischium) to form the hip joint (Figure 4.1). The head of the femur articulates with the pelvis at the acetabulum. The acetabulum of the pelvis is shallow at birth (3 degrees) and deepens over the course of the first 3 years (to 17 degrees) (Bernhardt 1988). The femur is relatively straight at birth with 150 degrees between the femoral shaft and neck in the coronal plane reducing to approximately 125 to 135 degrees by the age of 6 (Jordan et al. 1983). Maintenance of these neonatal values is one contributing factor of hip dislocation in children with cerebral palsy.

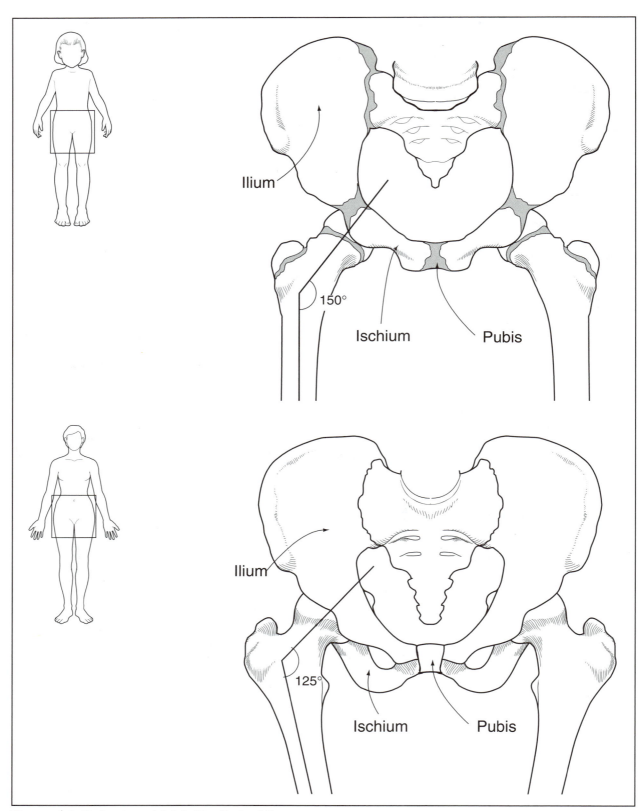

Figure 4.1. Pediatric and Adult Hip Skeletal Systems

At the hip, internal and external forces affect the joint's growth, development, and contribution to normal motor performance. The internal architecture of the femur forms by stress, with medial, lateral, and two accessory systems involved in the trabecular growth pattern. The medial trabecular system forms from the medial cortex of the femoral head radiating outward to the superior aspect of the femoral head, then down the medial shaft (Figure 4.2). This trabecular formation occurs along the lines of force in single limb stance (Singleton and Leveau 1975). The lateral trabecular system radiates from the lateral side of the upper femoral head to the inferior aspect of the head and across to the lateral aspect of the shaft. Abductor muscle pull and gravity appear to be responsible for the formation of this system (Radin et al. 1979; Singleton and Leveau 1975).

The sacroacetabular and the sacro-ischial trabecular systems of the pelvis transmit forces to the head of the femur and reinforce those areas receiving the most stress (Norkin and Levangie 1980).

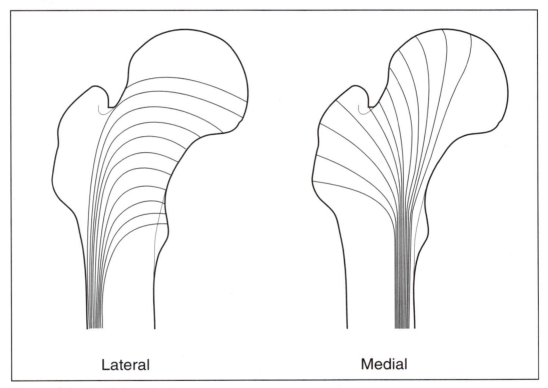

Lateral   Medial

Figure 4.2. Hip Trabecular System

Common Anomalies

Angle of Torsion

The angle of torsion is the angle the head of the femur makes with the condyles in a horizontal plane (Figure 4.3). It averages approximately 40 degrees of anterior torsion at birth (Badgley 1949; Beals 1969; Bleck 1982; Fabry et al. 1973; Hensinger and Jone 1982; Mattles 1965; McCrea 1985; Sutherland and Cooper 1984; Tachdjian 1971; Tax 1985), decreasing in the first two years to approximately 30 degrees (Bleck 1982; Engel and Staheli 1974; Fabry et al. 1973; Sutherland and Cooper 1984). This results in the characteristic frog-leg position of the infant. The residual amount of torsion, however, is variable up until 8 to 9 years of age, when the torsion approximates the adult norm of 12 to 15 degrees.

This bony angle influences the range of internal and external rotation available at the infant's hip. However, as the infant matures, relative rotation is variable, and this variability is used to assess relative ante- and retrotorsion (Haas et al. 1973; Hensinger and Jone 1982; Hoffer 1980; Phelps et al. 1985; Pitkow 1975; Tax 1985). If the infant hip is anteverted (i.e., angled forward more than 12 degrees), more internal rotation is naturally available, allowing the child to in-toe in standing and to reverse-tailor-sit. These positions are stable and do not cause other anomalies in the otherwise moving child. If the infant hip is retroverted (i.e., angled forward less than 12 degrees), more external rotation is naturally available, allowing the child to out-toe in standing and to tailor-sit comfortably. In standing, this torsion

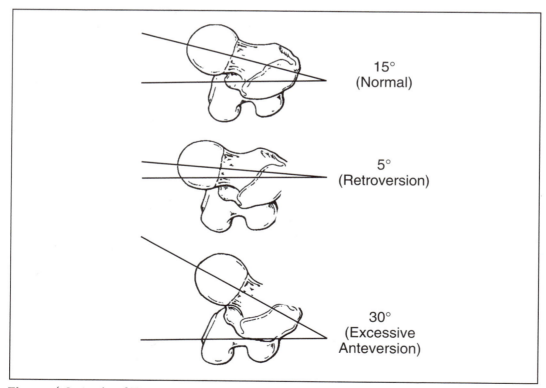

15°
(Normal)

5°
(Retroversion)

30°
(Excessive
Anteversion)

Figure 4.3. Angle of Torsion
Reproduced by permission of The Saunders Group, Inc. © 1996

influences the position of the hip and foot for stability. In antetorsion, because the femoral head must seat itself firmly in the acetabulum, and too much medial torsion occurs in the femur, the foot "toes in." This position would be the most stable for the child. Conversely, too much lateral torsion in the femur causes the foot to "toe out." Toeing in or out from excessive torsion is self-limiting but does take 8 to 9 years of growth to gradually improve in a normal child.

These naturally occurring hip positions must be considered when assessing the movement patterns of the child with neurological impairment. The child with antetorsion will in-toe and reverse tailor sit regardless of the therapeutic modalities used to treat the antetorsion. The antetorsion will not prevent the child from walking, nor necessarily cause knee pain from reverse-tailor-sitting, because children without neurological problems but with antetorsion have these same patterns. If there is a lack of external rotation for reasons other than bony alignment, however, this condition may be amenable to therapeutic intervention. Some of the causes of in-toeing that mimic antetorsion include hip capsular restriction, muscular imbalance, and bony anomalies in the tibia and forefoot.

To assess the cause of in-toeing, place the child prone. The hip must allow extension to at least neutral. If the hip does not have that much extension, the test for antetorsion is invalid as the other factors affecting in-toeing cannot be ruled out. Once the hip can be extended, flex the knee to 90 degrees and measure the relative amount of internal and external rotation. If the difference between the two ranges is greater than 10 degrees, the bone is twisted. Excess external rotation over internal rotation suggests the bone is retroverted. Excess internal rotation over external rotation suggests the bone is anteverted. However, if the ranges of internal and external rotation are within 10 degrees of each other, the in-toeing is not related to the torsion of the femur. Capsular limitations, muscular imbalance and other bony anomalies such as tibial torsion can then be assessed. Stuberg and Metcalf (1988) compared assessment of femoral torsion using goniometry and CAT scan, noting that the clinical assessment with the goniometer is by itself unreliable. Yet this clinical measure is the common assessment to determine recommendation of derotational osteotomies.

Angle of Inclination

The angle of inclination is the angle the femoral head makes with the shaft in a frontal plane (Figure 4.4). In infancy this angle is 150 degrees and gradually decreases to 120 degrees in the elderly. Maintenance of this angle beyond infancy is thought to contribute to the hip dislocations so often seen in children with cerebral palsy, and tends to cause the head of the femur to move superiorly and posteriorly. Any additional weight on the femur as well as pull of the muscle tends to force the femur farther superiorly and posteriorly. This angle changes due to the effects of weightbearing and the pull of the abductors. Therefore, intervention to develop a stable hip in the child with cerebral palsy should include standing with the weight through the femur and actively weightshifting. Note that neither of these can occur in a child with a 20-degree hip flexion contracture strapped into a forward- or backward-leaning standing frame. Loosening the straps so the child can wiggle slightly side-to-side and assuring adequate hip extension may assist in weight shifting necessary for remodeling the femur.

Though mobilization will not replace a dislocated hip, clinical experience suggests it can stop the progression of a subluxing hip, assist in preventing the malalignment in the first place, and provide necessary range for function even in a dislocated hip. Increasing the inferior extra-articular capsule flexibility can increase the abduction range available at the hip joint. Consequently, when the child stands, the weight goes through the femur, not at an angle to it. This changes the forces across the hip joint.

Newborn Hip Contracture and Mobilization

Capsular and muscular factors hold the newborn hip joint in a position of contracture. Therefore, extension of the hip joint is not a normal feature of the neonate (Bleck 1982; Haas et al. 1973; Hensinger and Jone 1982; Hoffer 1980; McCrea 1985; Sgarlato 1971). Lee's (1977) investigation of the cause of newborn hip contracture in stillborn infants revealed that capsular limitations, not physiologic flexion or muscle pull, caused hip contracture in the newborn.

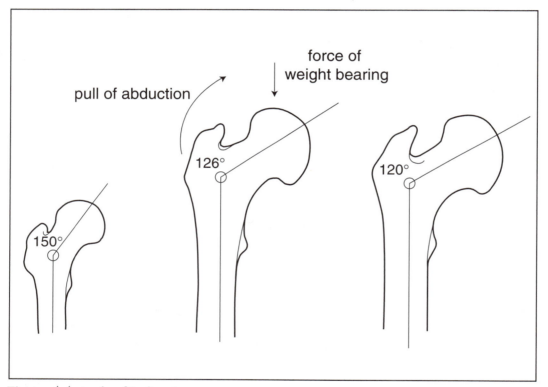

Figure 4.4. Angle of Inclination

Derotation of the femur and decrease in the contracture normally occur as hips are extended and externally rotated (Lee 1977) as infants achieve head up in prone or are supported in standing, and later when they stand on their own. This normal derotation does not occur in children with neurological dysfunction because they can not stretch their own extra-articular connective tissue due to their weakness. This manual suggests that joint mobilization techniques may be used to increase range of motion of joints abnormally limited by extra-articular connective tissue tightness, thus changing the placement of the center of gravity over the base of support, the force of gravity in weightbearing, and the line of muscle pull.

Joint mobility assessment must consider both range of motion and ligamentous flexibility. Any limitation to skeletal range of motion may have either bone or ligament causes. Range of motion is estimated or measured with a goniometer. Although adult range of motion values are well-documented, normal range of motion for some joints in infants (excluding the hip) have not been documented.

Activities of daily living seldom require full range of motion, but more range of motion is necessary for activities of daily living than for gait. The therapeutic community considers 90 degrees of hip flexion adequate for a child's sitting range. Unfortunately, this is not an adequate standard, for it will not allow a child to reach, feed, or dress with any sitting balance, as all those activities require the center of gravity to move forward and backward over the femurs in the reach. According to Johnston et al. (1970), 33 degrees of lateral rotation, 28 degrees of abduction and 124 degrees of flexion at the hip are needed for activities of daily living. Gait, on the other hand, only requires 10 degrees of hyperextension, 30 degrees of flexion, and 5 degrees of abduction. For example, many children with cerebral palsy sacral-sit because they lack 124 degrees of flexion and crouch-stand because they don't have 10 degrees of hyperextension. Total range of motion at the hip for children identified in the literature is reported in Table 4.1.

Ligamentous System

Ligaments support the articulations between the bones and limit joint motion. The three ligaments at the hip are named for the bones of the pelvis to which they attach: the ilio-, pubo-, and ischiofemoral (Figure 4.5). All three ligaments limit extension. Individual ligaments also limit other ranges (Kapandji 1970; Norkin and Levangie 1980). The iliofemoral ligament limits external rotation in conjunction with the pubofemoral ligament; the pubofemoral ligament limits abduction in extension and flexion greater than 90 degrees; and the ischiofemoral ligament limits internal rotation and extension (Kapandji 1970; Norkin and Levangie 1980). The position of maximum stability at the hip is therefore slight hyperextension, internal rotation, and adduction (as in single limb stance) when the ligaments are wound taut around the joint.

Table 4.1
Normal Hip Range of Motion Values for Children

Age	Motion	Range
0–3 months	Flexion*	120°
	Extension	–28° (range –20° to –60°)
	Internal rotation	60°
	External rotation	45° (range 25° –65°)
	Adduction	0°
3–6 months	Flexion	N.A.
	Extension	–7°
	Internal rotation	N.A.
	External rotation	87°
	Abduction	76°
	Adduction	N.A.
6–9 months	Flexion	N.A.
	Extension	N.A.
	Internal rotation	21°
	External rotation	45°
	Abduction	N.A.
	Adduction	N.A.
9–12 months	Flexion	N.A.
	Extension	–3°
	Internal rotation	N.A.
	External rotation	N.A.
	Abduction	59°
	Adduction	N.A.
18–36 months	Flexion	N.A.
	Extension	30°
	Internal rotation	N.A.
	External rotation	N.A.
	Abduction	45°
	Adduction	N.A.

*Using Staheli test method.

N.A. Not available.

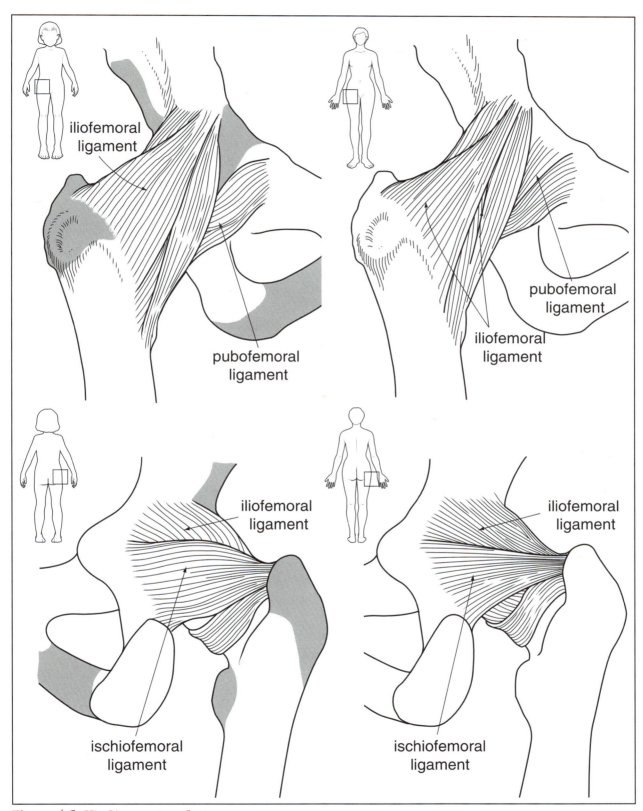

Figure 4.5. Hip Ligamentous System

Excessive tightness in these ligaments can produce characteristic limits to range of motion and movement patterns. The capsular pattern of restriction is characterized by maximum restriction in internal rotation and abduction with some restriction to flexion and extension. Children with neurological dysfunction frequently display this pattern. Therefore, assess and treat the tight connective tissue's contribution to the abnormal movement first; afterward, assess and treat the muscular and neurological causes for the motor dysfunction, if there are any.

Detecting Movement Patterns

Examining movement around each axis allows detection of movement patterns which may be frequently caused by ligamentous limitation. Efficient movement around a coronal axis requires full range of hip extension and flexion. The commonly seen anterior pelvic tilt in standing may be a lack of full hip extension, and posterior tilt in sitting may be a lack of flexion greater than 90 degrees. Without full hip joint flexibility, compensatory postures will occur in the spine and knees. For example, standing in an anterior pelvic tilt requires knee flexion and/or spinal extension to keep the head over the base of support. Otherwise, the child must hold a support as he or she cannot adjust the center of gravity over the base of support. Consequently, tightness in the anterior ligamentous support structures will limit extension at the hip, producing an apparent anterior pelvic tilt in the standing child. Tightness in the inferior ligamentous support structures of the hip joint will limit hip flexion greater than 90 degrees, resulting in apparent sacral-sitting in both long- and tailor-sitting positions.

Conversely, movement around a sagittal axis requires hip abduction and adduction. Limitation to the inferior hip ligamentous support structures limits free abduction in extension during swing phase necessary for correct foot placement at the beginning of stance phase, resulting in a tendency to adduct the leg, as in scissoring. Common substitutions include compensatory lateral trunk flexion or excessive hip adduction.

Movement around a vertical axis requires internal and external rotation of the hip. Limitation to the anterior periarticular connective tissue can prevent free external rotation of the swing leg during gait, resulting in an apparent in-toe gait. Compensatory rotation in the trunk and short stride length are common substitutions.

Stability in Stance

Stability at the hip joint in stance requires the coordination of several forces. These forces include position of the hip joint, gravity, and muscle pull. Changes in these forces applied early in reformation of a child's bone may affect the architecture of the bones.

In erect bilateral stance, the hip is slightly hyperextended and stable because the ligaments are taut in extension. Because gravity pulls the hip into extension, gravity assists to maintain the equilibrium around the hip when it is extended. Therefore, very little muscle activity is needed to maintain this position. If, however, the hip is flexed, significant muscle activity in the hamstrings and gluteals is required to maintain the position. This is consistent with the observation of chronically contracting hamstrings seen on EMG recordings of children with spastic diplegic cerebral palsy who frequently stand in hip flexion. EMGs simply signal muscle activity, not the cause of the activity. Although EMG recordings have been interpreted as suggesting spastic muscles, they may simply signal a muscle contracting correctly given the position of the center of gravity over the base of support.

Unilateral stance does require muscle action. Gravity tends to pull the pelvis down on the left when the body weight is transferred to the right leg. This pull must be counterbalanced by the gluteus medius on the right. This muscle requires significant strength to support the pelvis and left side of the body. If it is insufficient, the pelvis drops, producing either a positive Trendelenburg or the trunk laterally tilts producing a compensated Trendelenburg. These are frequently seen but not identified as such in children with cerebral palsy.

Assessment for ligamentous flexibility is measured by the joint play. Techniques to assess hip joint ligament flexibility are summarized in Table 4.2. Diagrams of the hand position and direction of force appear in Figures 4.6 and 4.7.

Table 4.2
Techniques to Assess Hip Joint Ligament Flexibility

Range	Technique	Hand Position	Force Direction
Extension	P–A glide	Stabilize the ASIS; mobilize the femoral head.	Femoral head moves anteriorly.
Flexion	Inferior glide	Stabilize the ASIS; mobilize the femoral head.	Femoral head moves inferiorly.
Abduction	Inferior glide	Stabilize the ASIS; mobilize the femoral head.	Femoral head moves inferiorly.
Adduction	Superior glide	Stabilize the ASIS; mobilize the femoral head.	Femoral head moves superiorly.
Internal rotation	A–P glide	Stabilize the ASIS; mobilize the femoral head.	Femoral head moves posteriorly.
External rotation	P–A glide	Stabilize the ASIS; mobilize the femoral head.	Femoral head moves anteriorly.

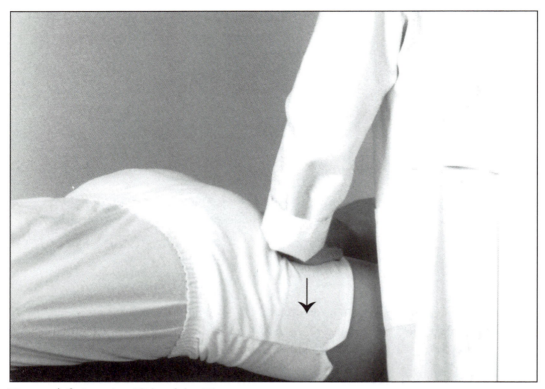

Figure 4.6. Anterior Glide of the Hip
Reproduced by permission of The Saunders Group, Inc. © 1996

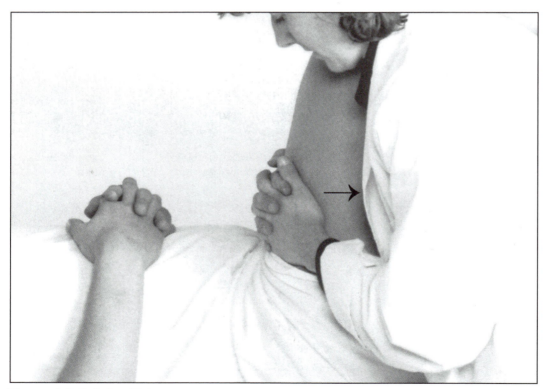

Figure 4.7. Inferior Glide
Reproduced by permission of The Saunders Group, Inc. © 1996

Muscular System

Infants cannot isolate muscles for classic muscle testing. However, determination of an individual muscle's flexibility, strength, or endurance is not the issue. The issue is the infant's ability to move the joint in any given direction without substitution.

Muscle flexibility testing for the infant must consider the rotational nature of the joint axis at the hip and the normal joint range of motion for the child's age. Table 4.3 describes muscle flexibility tests and substitutions.

Table 4.3
Hip Muscle Flexibility Testing for Children with Cerebral Palsy

Muscle Group	Testing Technique	Substitutions
Flexors:		
Iliopsoas	Position: Supine Stabilize: Pelvis Move: Femur Positive test: Femur does not fully extend at the hip to age-appropriate range. Similar pattern is seen in prone when child cannot fully extend hip through age-appropriate range of motion.	Limited hip joint flexibility, pelvis rocks forward, hips abduct/adduct, lumbar spine arches.
Quadriceps	Position: Supine Stabilize: Pelvis Move: Femur, knee flexed at 90°. Positive test: Hip does not fully extend and knee does not relax flexed at 90°. Similar pattern is seen in prone when child cannot fully extend hip and knee or when knee flexion requires corresponding hip flexion.	Hip joint limitation, knee joint limitation, pelvis rocks forward, hip abducts, lumbar spine arches.
Iliotibial	Position: Supine Stabilize: Pelvis Move: Femur into internal rotation and adduction with knee extended. Positive test: Limitation to full joint range. Similar pattern is seen in children post-adduction releases.	Hip joint limitation, knee joint limitation
Sartorius	Position: Supine Stabilize: Pelvis Move: Femur into external rotation and abduction with knee extended. Positive test: Limitation to full joint range.	Hip joint limitation, knee joint limitation
Extensors:		
Hamstrings	Position: Supine Stabilize: Pelvis and lumbar spine in flexion, either by firmly holding opposite leg down or by measuring hip range to the point where the pelvis rocks back as hip motion is completed. Move: Either the femur with knee straight (SLR) or flex the hip to 90° and extend the knee. Positive test: Hip flexion less than age-appropriate norm (SLR) or knee flexion less than age-appropriate norm. This is 70° in the adult and child. Ninety degrees is neither average in the normal population nor necessary for function—in long-sitting even normal adults sacral-sit.	Hip joint limitation, knee joint limitation, pelvic rotation, flexion of the other leg, pelvic tilt

Table 4.3
Hip Muscle Flexibility Testing for Children with Cerebral Palsy *(continued)*

Muscle Group	Testing Technique	Substitutions
Abductors:		
Gluteus medius	<u>Position</u>: Supine <u>Stabilize</u>: Pelvis <u>Move</u>: Femur into adduction and extension. <u>Positive test</u>: Hip joint does not move through full joint range.	Hip joint limitation, hip flexion
Adductors:		
Adductors	<u>Position</u>: Supine <u>Stabilize</u>: Pelvis <u>Move</u>: Femur into abduction with hip extension. <u>Positive test</u>: Hip joint does not move through the full joint range.	Hip joint limitation, hip flexion
Internal rotation	<u>Position</u>: Prone <u>Stabilize</u>: Pelvis <u>Move</u>: Flex knee, move tibia so femur internally rotates. <u>Positive test</u>: Internal rotation is more limited than explained by femoral torsion and joint capsule limitation.	Hip joint limitation, internal rotation limits
External rotation	<u>Position</u>: Prone <u>Stabilize</u>: Pelvis <u>Move</u>: Flex knee, move tibia so hip externally rotates. <u>Positive test</u>: External rotation is more limited than explained by femoral torsion and joint capsule limitation.	Hip joint limitation, external rotation limits

Hip muscle strength controls the placement of the center of gravity over the base of support in sitting and standing. Although it is easy to see hip strength in terms of leg movement on a fixed pelvis, balance in sitting and standing requires reverse action. That is, balance in sitting and standing requires that the hip muscles move the pelvis over fixed femurs. For example, the hamstrings extend the femur at the hip, but functionally they are critical for controlling the pelvis forward in sitting and standing. The resistance of upper extremity and trunk body weight in sitting balance is significantly greater than the resistance of the weight of the femur in hip extension. Consequently, just because the child can extend the hip by moving the femur from flexion to neutral that does not mean the hamstring is strong enough to control body weight when reaching forward in tailor-sitting. Treatment for weakness must address the appropriate amount of resistance in the appropriate range of motion for function. Table 4.4 presents a summary of proposed strength criteria for hip muscles.

Table 4.4
Proposed Strength Criteria for Hip Muscles

Strength Criteria	Iliopsoas	Quadriceps	Gluteals	Hamstrings	Abductors	Adductors
Poor (Movement with gravity eliminated.)	Pulls femur all the way to chest in prone in preparation for crawling or rolling.	As with iliopsoas for rectus, knee extension along the floor.	In sidelying, will child extend through the available range?	As with gluteals, but with knee extended.	Abducts legs in prone, as in preparation to crawl or sit.	Can bring legs together on the support.
Fair (Movement full range against gravity.)	Can bring knee to chest against gravity in supine, or in sitting, can kick so that femur moves up to chest.	Full knee extension antigravity kick, otherwise as with iliopsoas.	Prone "swimming" or Landau reaction.	As with gluteals, but with knee extended.	Sidestepping.	Can kick leg across midline in slight hip flexion.
Good (Movement against gravity and some resistance.)	Can raise femur to chest against some resistance, i.e., weight of shoes.	Full knee extension antigravity with shoes, otherwise as with iliopsoas.	As above, but with resistance, such as shoes or toys.	As with gluteals, but with knee extended.	Sidestepping with resistance such as shoes or single limb stance with pelvis level.	Can kick leg across midline against resistance, i.e., a soccer ball.
Normal (Age-appropriate resistance.)	Can raise femur to chest against age-appropriate resistance.	—	—	—	—	Can kick leg across midline against age appropriate resistance.
At 3 months	Crawling movements.	Leg thrusts in play.	Swims	—	Thrusts leg in play, holds leg up.	
At 6 months	Stepping movements.	Early stepping movements.		Sits alone momentarily.	Balances in sitting, playing to one side.	
At 9 months	Leg up in pull-to-stand.	Pulls to stand.	Shifts weight while standing, extending hip.	Moves from sitting to creeping.	Cruises sideways.	
At 12 months	Walking	Sits down with control.	Walks backward.	Sits down.	Raises to stand, one leg up.	Walking.
At 18 months	Walks up stairs with help.	Walks steps with help, especially down.	Walking.	Squats.		
At 24 months	Marks time on stairs independently.	Jumps off floor.	Stands on one foot with help.		Stands on one foot.	Stands on one foot.
At 36 months	Alternates feet on steps, independently kicks a ball.	Distance jump at least 4 inches.	Ascends/descends stairs, alternating feet.	Hops.	Kicks ball.	Stands on one foot.

Treatment Planning

Any assessment must determine functional strengths and weaknesses and the specific proximate causes of those weaknesses. Differentiation of each problem's proximate cause is critical for effective and efficient treatment. Once causal factors are tested, identified, and ruled out (capsular first, then bony, muscular, and finally neurological), a treatment plan can be developed. For example, in-toeing may be due to femoral torsion, capsular tightness, or muscle weakness. In a normal child, femoral torsion is monitored; however, a child with cerebral palsy may receive a derotational osteotomy. If capsular tightness is suspected, mobilization is indicated. If weakness is presumed to be the cause, strengthening is prescribed. If synergies are implicated, inhibition or other neurological approaches are the preferred intervention strategies. This approach can be applied to three common motor problems for children with cerebral palsy: sacral-sitting, crouch standing and decreased stride length.

Sacral-Sitting

Sacral-sitting is the posture assumed by children with cerebral palsy during long-sitting and frequently in tailor-sitting. The child sits with the center of gravity too far posterior to the hip joint, resulting in a posterior pelvic tilt and a rounded back. Although limitation of hamstring flexibility is assumed to be the cause of sacral-sitting, its contribution can be ruled out easily. Simply flex the child's knees so the child is tailor-sitting. Children with cerebral palsy, even in tailor-sitting, frequently cannot bring the pelvis forward over the femurs to 120 degrees of hip flexion. Hence, many children with cerebral palsy who tailor-sit still do so with a posterior pelvic tilt, producing an inability to shift the center of gravity forward for reaching, yet the hamstrings cannot be the cause. This same limitation to hip flexion interferes in reach for the child in bench-sitting. While bench-sitting, sacral-sitting appears to be reduced because the pelvis is vertical. However, the pelvis still cannot move forward over the fixed femurs allowing reach for many children with cerebral palsy. The inability to shift the pelvis forward over the femurs is very apparent in children sitting at a 90 degree seat angle in a wheelchair when they have less than 90 degrees of hip flexion. This problem frequently results in difficulty positioning children in 90-degree wheelchairs, or the boomerang effect when the wheelchair's seat belt is released.

Once the range of motion is present, the muscular system can be assessed. Once the range is achieved for children who sacral-sit, they may be placed in ring-sitting position, but they may be unable to balance or use their upper extremities while sitting. Balance in ring-sitting requires hamstring strength eccentrically and concentrically against resistance of the trunk at 90 to 125 degrees of hip flexion. Additional resistance to the muscle occurs when the arms reach forward or the hands manipulate a toy. Once the strength in the correct type of contraction in the correct part of the range is achieved, then neurological considerations of speed, coordination, and motor planning can be addressed therapeutically.

Table 4.5 lists some of the possible causes and treatment options for the child who sacral-sits.

Table 4.5
Common Evaluation Results and Treatment Options for Sacral-Sitting

System	Findings	Treatment Options
Skeletal	Limitation in hip flexion range less than 120°.	Mobilize hip inferiorly until at least 120° of flexion range is available.
	Fixed hip contracture.	Adjust seating system to child's fixed range.
	Lumbar flexion.	Mobilize lumbar spine anteriorly.
Muscular	Hamstring flexibility (seldom the cause).	Muscle stretching, casting, or lengthening.
	Hamstring weakness (frequently a contributing factor).	Strengthen hamstrings eccentrically and concentrically between 90° and 120° of hip flexion against resistance of trunk, arms and toys.
	Hip flexor weakness eccentrically and concentrically.	Strengthen hip flexors eccentrically and concentrically between 70° and 90° of hip flexion against resistance of trunk, arms and toys.
	Back extensor weakness.	Strengthen back extensors eccentrically and concentrically between full flexion and extension.
	Poor muscular endurance.	Train for endurance in this hip and back range of motion.
Nervous	Decreased rapid alternating movements.	Move between 80° and 100° of flexion, increasing speed of oscillation at hip.
	Weakness due to neurological damage, peripherally or centrally.	Adapt environment around need of child.
	Documented damage to the vestibular system.	Focus child on other sources of proprioceptive input or adapt environment around child.

Crouch Standing

Children with spastic diplegic cerebral palsy frequently crouch-stand. Crouch standing requires considerable energy and muscular effort to support poorly aligned joints and includes lumbar flexion, hip flexion, knee flexion, and either excessive ankle dorsiflexion or plantarflexion with transverse tarsal malalignment. Hamstrings and adductors contract to support the hip, quadriceps contract to support the knee, and the gastrocsoleous contracts to support the ankle isometrically. These muscle contractions mimic increased tone. However, the contractions may not be a result of increased tone but the normal actions of the muscles to the abnormal joint range limiting the placement of the center of gravity over the base of support. Because they are supporting the skeleton, the muscles cannot efficiently ambulate the body. Often tight hamstrings are assumed to be the only cause when, in fact, there are many reasons for crouch standing (Table 4.6).

Table 4.6
Common Evaluation Results and Treatment Options
for the Hip in Crouch Standing

System	Findings	Treatment Options
Skeletal	Limited hip extension — less than 10° of hyperextension	Mobilize hip anteriorly.
	Limited knee extension	Mobilize knee anteriorly or externally as appropriate to contracture.
	Limited ankle and foot range	Mobilize ankle/foot joints as appropriate to contractures.
	Excessive ankle and foot range	Stabilize ankle/foot with orthotic or surgery.
	Fixed contractures	Adjust environment to child's needs.
Muscular	Limited hip flexors and extensors; ankle musculature	Stretch, cast, or surgery.
	Weakness of hip extensors, hip flexors, knee extensors, knee flexors, and ankle dorsi- or plantarflexors	Strengthen muscles eccentrically and concentrically between 80° of hip flexion and 5° of hip hyperextension, between 5° of flexion and full extension at the knee, and between 10° of plantarflexion and 5° of dorsiflexion at the ankle.
	Poor endurance of back, hip, knee and ankle muscles	Train for endurance of these muscles in this range.
Nervous	Decreased rapid alternating movements	Rapidly contract/relax muscles in range noted above.
	Peripheral or central induced weakness	Adapt environment to child.
	Documented damage to the vestibular system	Adapt environment to child.

Before one can say the hamstrings are contracting abnormally due to spasticity or brain damage, hip extension must be available. If placing a child in full hip extension antigravity doesn't stop the contraction of the hamstrings, then they may be a cause of the motor dysfunction. However, if placing the child in full hip extension stops contraction of the hamstrings, the joint contracture is a cause of the crouch-standing posture whereas the muscle action is a normal response to the center of gravity over the base of support. Next, assess the contribution of the muscular system. For example, in the child who can now achieve hip extension but keeps collapsing back to a crouch-standing posture, weakness of the hip flexors and extensors eccentrically and concentrically between 5 degrees of hyper-extension and 5 degrees of flexion may prevent the child from controlling the center of gravity over the base of support when swaying or initiating a step.

Remember, any given child could have one, some, or all of the above causes, requiring an individualized specific treatment program.

Decreased Stride Length

Decreased stride length during gait is characteristic of many children with cerebral palsy. Again, hamstring length is frequently implicated as a causative factor for decreased gait efficiency, but many other factors must be ruled out prior to surgical lengthening of the muscles. Table 4.7 lists some of those causes and treatment options.

Table 4.7
**Common Evaluation Results and Treatment Options
for the Hip in Decreased Stride Length**

System	Findings	Treatment Options
Skeletal	Limited hip hyperextension	Mobilize hip anteriorly.
	Limited sacral rotation	Mobilize sacroiliac joint.
	Limited back extension	Mobilize lumbar spine anteriorly.
Muscular	Limited hamstring flexibility (infrequently the case)	Stretch, cast, or lengthen.
	Limited hip flexor flexibility	Stretch, cast, or lengthen.
	Weak hip flexors	Strengthen flexors eccentrically into hyperextension.
	Weak quadriceps	Strengthen quadriceps concentrically through the range, especially at terminal knee extension.
	Weak gastrocsoleous	Strengthen ankle eccentrically through the range.
	Decreased endurance	Train for endurance.
Nervous	Poor rapid alternating movements	Oscillate hip, knee, and ankle in and out of close-pack positions.
	Weakness from central or peripheral neuropathy	Adapt environment to child.

Summary

Hip joint mobility is critical to control the center of gravity over the base of support. Placement of the center of gravity relative to the base of support normally determines which muscles are necessary to move in space. Any limitation to hip joint mobility will result in movement patterns commonly exhibited by children with cerebral palsy. Only after removing the contribution of the hip joint limitation to motor performance can a therapist address and assess the contribution of muscle weakness, flexibility, and poor endurance to the poor motor performance. After that, a therapist can assess and address motor planning, speed of response, rapid alternating movements and other neural considerations.

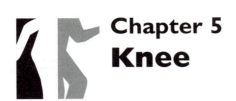

Chapter 5
Knee

The knee joint adjusts leg length during stance phase of gait and controls the excursion of the center of gravity over the base of support. It also responds to the positions of the hip and ankle-foot complex. Therefore, hip flexion contractures place excess stress on the femoral-tibial articulation, excess pressure on the patellar articulating surface, and excess demands on the strength of the quadriceps. Malalignment of the ankle-foot complex often stresses the knee more on one side than the other. All of these excess stresses force the knee to flex or hyperextend to control the center of gravity over the base of support.

Skeletal System

Bones of the knee joint are the femur, patella, and the tibia (Figure 5.1). The tibiofemoral and patellofemoral joints are maintained within the same capsule, but move very differently. Common variations in the bones include the tibiofemoral joint angle and tibial torsion.

The articulation of the femur and the tibia forms an angle known as physiologic valgus. The infant has no angle between these bones. Physiologic valgus at the knee forms as the femoral angle of inclination decreases, bringing the distal end of the femur in toward the midline. This change in relationship between the femur and the tibia has the effect of narrowing the base of support and decreasing the excursion of the center of gravity over the base of support in gait. Normal angle develops to between 165 and 170 degrees (increase in the angle is genu varum, decrease is genu valgum).

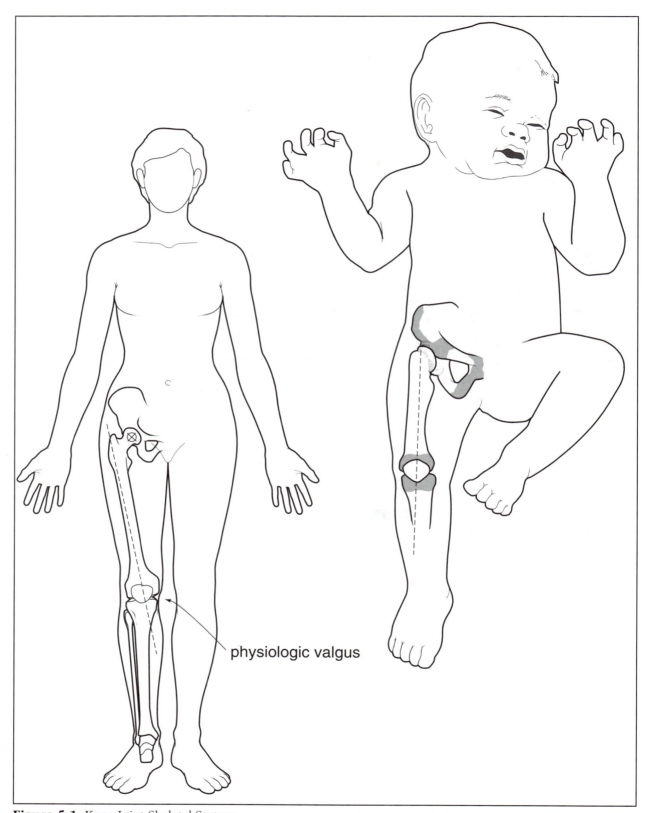

physiologic valgus

Figure 5.1. Knee Joint Skeletal System

As with the femur, the tibia is twisted through the shaft, showing varying degrees of torsion. To test for the torsion, line the tibial tuberosity up until it is perpendicular to the support. A line through the malleoli intersecting the support forms the angle of torsion (Figure 5.2). The average torsion in the adult is between 15 and 30 degrees of an external twist. Children are much more variable, and the variability gradually decreases until age 8. Torsion greater than 30 degrees outward is external tibial torsion, but torsion less than 15 degrees outward is internal tibial torsion. This line through the malleoli is also the axis of the talocrural joint, and it determines the direction of the tibia's forward movement over the talus during gait. The angle in turn affects foot placement in stance.

Table 5.1
Combinations of Femoral and Tibial Torsions with Resultant Foot Placement

Femur	Tibia	Foot Placement
Anteversion	Internal tibial torsion	Foot toes in.
Anteversion	External tibial torsion	Depends on relative amount of torsion.
Retroversion	Internal tibial torsion	Depends on relative amount of torsion.
Retroversion	External tibial torsion	Foot toes out.
Normal	Internal tibial torsion	Foot toes in.
Normal	External tibial torsion	Foot toes out.
Anteversion	Normal	Foot toes in.
Retroversion	Normal	Foot toes out.
Normal	Normal	Foot toes slightly out.

Joint Motion

Address joint motion only after determining bone alignment. Flexion motion from full extension to 15 degrees of flexion is internal rotation of the tibia on the femur. Flexion beyond 15 degrees is primarily sliding of the tibia on the femur in non-weightbearing or femur on tibia in weightbearing (Wisman et al. 1980). Therefore, flexion is a combination of femoral posterior roll and anterior glide, or tibial posterior roll and posterior glide on the femur. Conversely, extension is a combination of femoral anterior roll and posterior glide.

Terminal knee extension consists of roll and spin such that the femur moves medially on the tibia to lock the joint during weightbearing while the tibia glides laterally in non-weight-bearing to lock the knee. Flexion of the knee requires unlocking of the joint, including lateral rotation of the femur on the tibia in weightbearing and medial rotation of the tibia on the femur in non-weightbearing loads. On a fixed tibia (as in moving from stand-to-sit), the femur rolls externally to move from full extension to 15 degrees of flexion. It then glides forward and rolls back from 15 degrees of flexion to full flexion. This pattern is reversed in moving from flexion to extension (as in sit-to-stand). When the femur is fixed (as in sitting while swinging the lower leg), the tibia unlocks the knee in extension by rolling internally. The tibia glides down and back on the femur for flexion greater than 15 degrees and is reversed as the tibia swings back into extension.

Children with cerebral palsy often have difficulty achieving full extension range because the rotary component of this locking mechanism is frequently missing. A child who cannot use the ligamentous knee-locking mechanism must rely on the bones as in genu recurvatum or the muscles as in flexed knee stance. Either strategy puts undue stress on the articular surfaces or the muscles.

Free motion of the patella is necessary for full tibiofemoral joint motion. The patella acts as a sesamoid bone, increasing the movement arm of the quadriceps through the range. Without the patella, as when it is riding too high on the femur in patella alta, the line of pull of the quadriceps approximates the axis of the femur. The parallel axis does not create the lever arm necessary for the quadriceps to move the tibia. Even if the quadriceps have normal strength, they would be unable to move the tibia effectively without the lever created by the patella. Children with cerebral palsy are doubly disadvantaged if the patella rides high on the femur, because this prevents the often weak quadriceps from supporting their body weight in crouch standing. This may be one reason why so many children with cerebral palsy who stand in a flexed posture give up standing and walking by their teenage years.

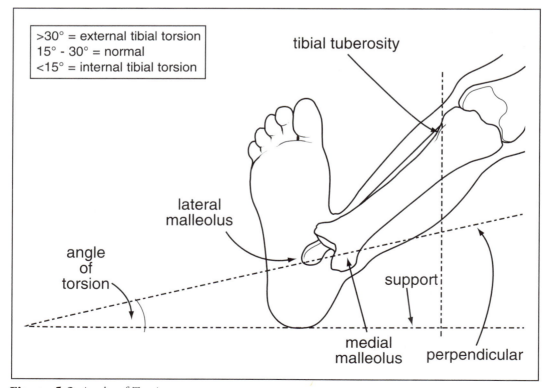

Figure 5.2. Angle of Torsion

A patella femoral grinding test gives an indication of the quality of the articular surfaces between the patella and the femur. These surfaces frequently are roughened and painful in degenerative changes and chondromalacia patellae. It is common for older children with cerebral palsy to develop knee pain; even though the movement disorder can be addressed from a neurological perspective, the pain must be approached from an acute orthopedic perspective.

Knee joint range of motion develops at the same time as hamstring flexibility. Term newborns are frequently born with 20 to 27 degrees of knee flexion contractures (Frankel 1973). To differentiate hamstring and joint limitation, Frankel extended the knee with the hamstring on slack (hip relatively extended), noting the joint limitation. Then he used the straight leg raise test to assess hamstring flexibility. He found that the joint and muscle flexibility appeared together by age 8 months (Frankel 1973). Table 5.2 lists normal range of motion values identified in the literature.

Table 5.2
Normal Knee Range of Motion Values for Children

Age	Motion	Range	Test Method
0–3 months	Flexion	135°	
	Extension	Popliteal angle contracture and connective tissue contracture with hip relatively extended 20°–30°.	Popliteal angle
3–6 months	Flexion	135°	
	Extension	Popliteal angle contracture and connective tissue contracture with hip relatively extended.	Popliteal angle
6–9 months	Flexion	135°	
	Extension	0° full hamstring flexibility and full knee joint range is present by 8 months.	Popliteal angle
18–36 months	Flexion	120°–130°	Prone with knee flexed.
	Extension	0°	
	Internal rotation	30° at 90° of flexion, 0° at full extension.	
	External rotation	40° at 90° of flexion, 0° at full extension.	

Frankel's technique can be applied to assessing the proximate cause of knee flexion contracture in children with neurological involvement because it is critical to differentiate between joint and muscular limitation in the child with cerebral palsy, as the treatment options for the two problems are completely different. Classical diagnosis requires extension of the limb and firm pressure on the anterior aspect of the knee joint. If the knee joint fails to extend to the zero position, then a joint flexion contracture is present (Bleck 1987). This joint contracture must be ruled out before assessing hamstring flexibility because a capsular limitation at the knee joint prevents full range of the joint during muscle flexibility testing, thereby preventing a diagnosis of muscle contracture.

Tardieu (1987) considered 20 degrees of popliteal angle as normal in the newborn. Johnson and Ashurst (1989) assessed popliteal angle as a predictor of cerebral palsy, suggesting the possibility that abnormal range of motion identified early in development might be useful in predicting abnormally developing children. At 7 to 8 months of age, when most of the infants were tested, 24 percent of infants born at less than 30 weeks of gestation had greater than a 10 degree popliteal angle. However, only 7 percent of infants born after more than 37 weeks of gestation had greater than a 10 degree angle. If children had less than a 10-degree popliteal angle at 7 to 8 months of age, they did not display cerebral palsy later. Of the children with more than a 10-degree angle, 12 percent had cerebral palsy whereas another 13 percent had other problems. In other words, decreased range of motion identified a population at risk for later problems. This may be the source of the very common 20-degree knee flexion contracture in older children with cerebral palsy. The child simply never stretched out the normal newborn contracture.

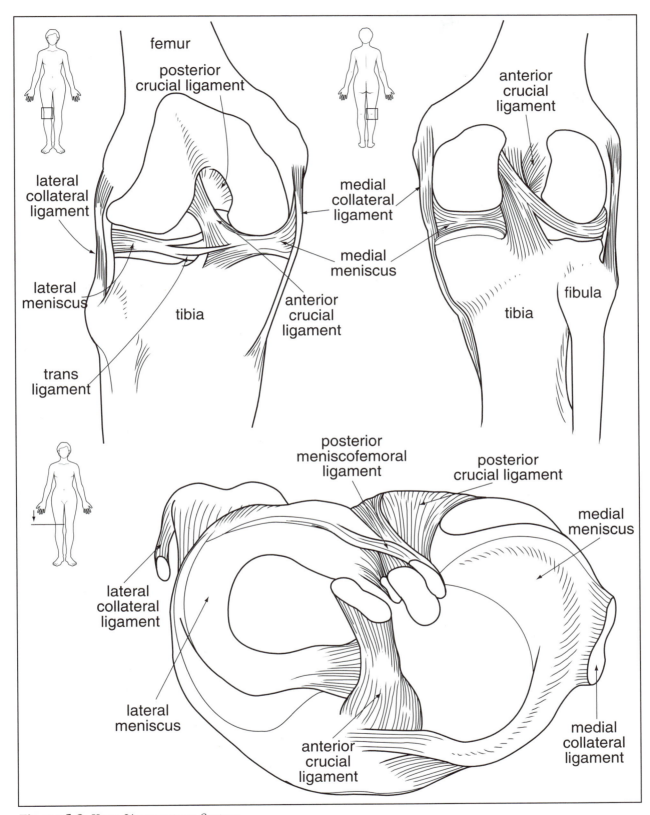

femur

posterior
crucial ligament

anterior
crucial
ligament

lateral
collateral
ligament

medial
collateral
ligament

medial
meniscus

lateral
meniscus

anterior
crucial
ligament

tibia

fibula

tibia

trans
ligament

posterior
meniscofemoral
ligament

posterior
crucial ligament

medial
meniscus

lateral
collateral
ligament

lateral
meniscus

anterior
crucial
ligament

medial
collateral
ligament

Figure 5.3. Knee Ligamentous System

Ligamentous System

The menisci are attached to the joint capsule by coronary ligaments, to the condyles by the meniscofemoral and meniscotibial ligaments, and to each other by the transverse ligament. The menisci act as the joint's shock absorbers, improve stability by deepening the articular surface, and improve mobility by reducing friction between the bones. The medial meniscus also attaches to the medial collateral ligament, and the lateral meniscus also attaches to the lateral collateral ligament. Medial and lateral collateral ligaments provide lateral stability, whereas the anterior and posterior cruciates control the slide of the femur on the tibia. See Figure 5.3 for the relationships between bones and ligaments.

To assess the knee joint ligaments for anterior/posterior joint stability, stabilize the femur. Grasp the tibia and push (pull) posteriorly (anteriorly) (Figure 5.4). There should be very little joint play. Children with cerebral palsy, especially children who stand in recurvatum, frequently show excessive laxity in these ligaments. Unfortunately, once they are stretched, very little can be done to return the ligaments to their normal tensile strength.

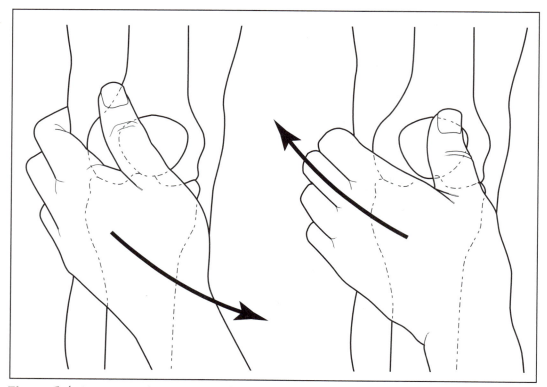

Figure 5.4. Anterior and Posterior Glide

Besides testing for anterior and posterior stability, check the medial and lateral collateral ligaments for stability (Figure 5.5). Extend the knee, stabilize the femur, and tip the tibia laterally or medially to determine the integrity of the ligaments. Excessive laxity can be related to knee joint pain, attempts to stabilize the joint with excessive muscle force, or avoidance of certain positions of the knee. Next, assess the rotary integrity of the tibia on the femur (Figure 5.6). Stabilize the femur with the knee joint at 90 degrees of flexion. Grasp the tibia at the malleoli and twist it medially or laterally. At 90 degrees of flexion, rotation should be free. This ligamentous flexibility is required for the joint to lock correctly in extension.

Any limitation to the flexibility of the ligaments limits full extension. Because the ligaments are normally taut in relative extension, any unusual tightness would limit the excursion to that range, producing a flexion contracture. Assess the capsular or ligamentous limit to normal motion by lying the child with cerebral palsy supine. In this position, the hamstrings are relatively slack because the hip is relatively extended. If the knee does not fully extend, the ligaments must be at least one of the limiting tissues (Bleck 1987; Rang et al. 1986). Muscle length is implicated as a causal factor in knee contracture only when the knee joint demonstrates full range when the hamstrings are on slack and subsequent muscle flexibility tests implicate the hamstrings. Table 5.3 lists techniques to test knee ligament flexibility.

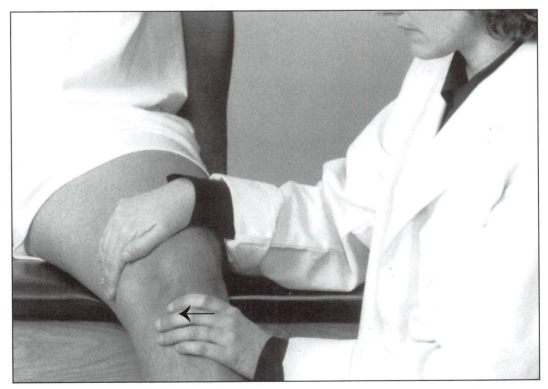

Figure 5.5. Medial Tilt
Reproduced by permission of The Saunders Group, Inc. © 1996

Table 5.3
Techniques to Assess Knee Ligament Flexibility

Range	Technique	Hand Position	Force Direction
Flexion:			
From −15° to full flexion	P-A glide post drawer sign	Stabilize the femur and mobilize the tibia.	Tibia moves posteriorly.
From full extension to 15°	Internal rotation	Stabilize the femur and mobilize the tibia.	Tibia moves internally.
Extension:			
From full flexion to −15°	A-P glide anterior drawer sign	Stabilize the femur and mobilize the tibia.	Tibia moves anteriorly.
From −15° to 0°	External rotation	Stabilize the femur and mobilize the tibia.	Tibia moves externally.

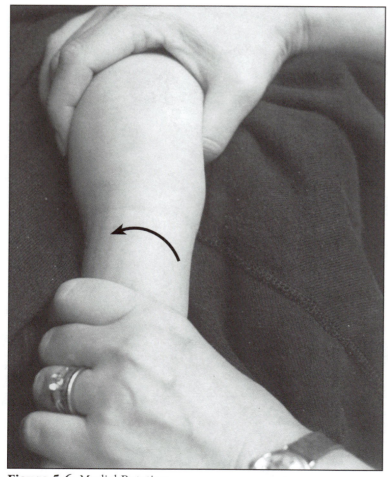

Figure 5.6. Medial Rotation

Muscular System

The knee flexors are the semitendinosus, semimembranosus, and the biceps femoris (hamstrings), sartorius (forming the pes anserinus with the semitendinosus and gracilis tendons), gracilis, popliteus, and the gastrocnemius. The knee extensors are the quadriceps femoris including the rectus, vastus intermedius, vastus lateralis, and vastus medialis.

Assessing Flexibility

Flexibility is the first variable in muscular assessment at the knee. Because limited muscular flexibility can mimic neurological synergy, inaccurate assessment and treatment result. For example, a tight rectus femoris often appears when the child with cerebral palsy is prone and the knee is flexed. Tightness in the rectus femoris causes hip flexion when flexing the knee. This pattern is often identified as a neurological reflex or synergy requiring a neurological treatment approach. Although this interpretation is a possibility, the muscle tightness can readily be ruled out. If stretching the rectus to normal flexibility (as assessed in supine) makes hip flexion disappear when the knee is flexed in prone, the motor pattern is due to a tight muscle and not a reflex. However, if the rectus has full flexibility as measured in the supine test and the motor pattern remains, then there is a neurological cause. These two examples clearly illustrate the multiple possible causes for a given motor pattern. A sequential assessment and treatment scheme designed to rule out some of the multiple causes of the motor problem may allow effective therapy to documentable problems.

Table 5.4 lists techniques to assess muscle flexibility.

Table 5.4
Knee Muscle Flexibility Testing for Children with Cerebral Palsy

Muscle Group	Testing Technique	Substitutions
Hamstrings	Popliteal angle: Stabilize the pelvis, flex the femur to 90°, and extend knee to full range.	Knee flexion contracture due to connective tissue limitation, full extension of the knee with 90° flexion of hip is not normal.
Quadriceps	Prone: With hip extended, flex knee to 90°; flexion of hip upon flexion of knee suggests short rectus femoris.	Positive test mimics neurological synergy pattern; the patterns are implicated only when full flexibility is present.

Assessing Strength

Strength is the second variable to consider in the muscular assessment of the knee. The quadriceps femoris normally acts at the knee eccentrically to control flexion and concentrically to control extension during closed kinematic chain activities (i.e., sitting, standing, or motion over the support leg in gait). Children with cerebral palsy who lack terminal knee extensor strength in concentric and eccentric contractions often avoid the knee flexion phase of stance (0 to 5 degrees of knee flexion) by hyperextending the knee or remaining crouched at 20 degrees of knee flexion.

Maintenance of the flexed knee posture requires continuous quadriceps and hamstring activity. In full extension, the extensor muscles are not necessary to maintain the knee position because the center of gravity is anterior to the axis of the knee tending to hold the joint in extension. The support structures of the back of the knee normally prevent hyperextension in standing. The child with cerebral palsy often cannot achieve a close-packed position of knee extension and requires isometric quadriceps to maintain the position. To decrease the muscular work, an alternate strategy to support the knee is genu recurvatum. No muscular effort is required as the overstretched ligaments allow bone support.

The knee flexion phase of gait requires concentric and eccentric contraction of the quadriceps to control the knee between 10 degrees of flexion and full extension while supporting the body. Children with cerebral palsy frequently have weakness in this range of motion and have two available compensating strategies. Either they avoid that range of knee flexion altogether by ambulating with excessive knee flexion, as in crouch gait, or they snap the joint through the range and lock it in recurvatum. Either strategy lowers the center of gravity, decreases the need for the concentric and eccentric contractions of the quadriceps, and puts additional stress on the bony and ligamentous structures of the joint to compensate.

The hamstrings limit excessive extension at the knee by decelerating the knee in the swing phase of gait. This eccentric contraction of the hamstrings is frequently missing in the child with cerebral palsy as the hamstrings are isometrically contracting to hold the flexed hip up against gravity. Therefore, many children with cerebral palsy can contract the hamstrings, but they are unable to use them in the coordinated manner required for efficient gait.

Table 5.5 lists suggested criteria for muscle strength assessment at the knee.

Table 5.5
Proposed Strength Criteria for Knee Muscles

Strength Criteria	Flexors	Extensors
Poor (Movement with gravity eliminated)	Sidelying, knee flexion	Knee extension through available range in sidelying.
Fair (Movement full range against gravity)	Prone, knee flexion	Knee extension through available range in supine.
Good (Movement against gravity and some resistance)	Prone, knee flexion with resistance such as shoes	Knee extension through available range in supine with some resistance, i.e., shoes.
Normal (Age-appropriate resistance)	Prone, knee flexion with age-appropriate resistance	Knee extension through available range in supine with age-appropriate resistance.
At 3 months	Prone kicking	Thrusts legs and holds them up.
At 6 months	N.A.	N.A.
At 9 months	Gets to sitting from prone (acts at pelvis), moves from sitting to creeping.	Bounces while supporting weight, shifts weight while standing, pulls to stand.
At 12 months	Walks alone (decelerating swing of tibia).	Sits down.
At 18 months	N.A.	N.A.
At 24 months	Ascends and descends stairs.	Jumps off floor.
At 36 months	Decelerating tibia in kicking	Ascends and descends stairs.

N.A. Not available

Assessing Endurance

Endurance is the third variable to consider in the muscular assessment at the knee. Given the speed with which a child ambulates, muscles must quickly contract and relax repetitively. Frequently, children with cerebral palsy can produce the desired contractions and relaxations when ambulating slowly or for short distances, but cannot maintain them when ambulating at a comfortable and functional speed. Both the neurological damage itself and poor muscular endurance can present this motor symptom. A training program may have a functional and measurable effect on the muscular endurance and distance ambulated.

Treatment Planning

Common motor problems in children with cerebral palsy affecting the knee include crouch gait and genu recurvatum.

Crouch Gait

Crouch gait in standing and walking is a common clinical problem for the therapist. The position puts undue stress on the knee, often resulting in patella alta or chondromalacia patellae. Crouch position may be caused by a variety of range and strength problems at the hip, knee, and ankle (see Table 5.6).

A lack of hip extension requires either knee flexion or genu recurvatum to compensate and allow the head to remain over the base of support. Malalignment of the foot joints can have the same effect. Also, of course, the knee joint itself may have an extra-articular tissue contracture as well.

Weakness in the quadriceps in terminal knee extension with isometric strength in the quadriceps at 20 degrees of knee flexion may cause the child with cerebral palsy to maintain a crouch position even when appropriate range exists at all joints. Alternately, the child with cerebral palsy may bypass the quadriceps weakness completely by snapping the knee into recurvatum.

Genu recurvatum (Hyperextension)

Genu recurvatum in children with cerebral palsy is frequently a subluxation of the tibia on the femur, as opposed to excessive extension utilizing the external rotation necessary in the knee locking mechanism. Management of the problem is dependent upon the contribution of all the joints in the lower extremities. The best management is prevention; once the support structures of the knee are overstretched, they seldom return to normal.

Table 5.6 lists common factors and treatment options in hypertension.

Table 5.6
Common Evaluation Results and Treatment Options in Knee Hyperextension

System	Findings	Treatment Options
Skeletal	Hip joint contracture	Mobilize support structures
	Knee joint hypermobility	Brace
	No terminal knee rotation	Mobilize tibia into external rotation
	Ankle joint contracture	Mobilize talocrural joint
Muscular	Hip muscle contracture	Stretch or lengthen flexors
	Weak quadriceps	Strengthen quadriceps in terminal extension concentrically and eccentrically
	Weak hamstrings	Strengthen hamstrings eccentrically against the resistance of a swinging tibia
	Weak gastrocsoleous	Strengthen gastrocsoleous eccentrically against body weight, as in moving from initial contact to midstance

Summary

Limited or excessive range of motion and weakness at any one joint requires compensation by the others in a closed kinematic chain. The knee responds to forces from both the hip and foot. Generally, each child with cerebral palsy displays motor performance problems due to combinations of joint limitations and muscle weakness. The combination unique to that child, when properly assessed, leads directly to the criteria necessary for effective and efficient multisystem treatment techniques.

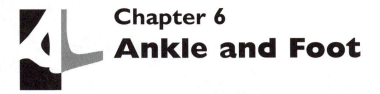

Chapter 6
Ankle and Foot

The foot stabilizes and mobilizes. As a stabilizer, it functions first as a base of support, and second as a rigid lever for push-off. As a mobilizer, it absorbs the rotary stress imposed by more proximal joints. To fulfill these functions, the foot has three primary joints: the talocrural, the subtalor, and the transverse tarsal joints.

Skeletal System

The bones of the foot and ankle can be grouped by joint:

talocrural joint	talus, tibia, and fibula
subtalor joint	talus and calcaneus
midtarsal joint	subtalor joint plus the cuboid and navicular
tarsometatarsal joints	3 cuneiforms and 5 metatarsals
metatarsal phalangeal joints	5 metatarsals and 5 phalanxes

Figure 6.1 shows the anatomical arrangement.

The axis of the ankle or talocrural joint determines foot position and the direction of weight shifted in forward propulsion. A normal adult axis at the talocrural joint faces 15 to 30 degrees externally. In children, however, the axis is considerably more variable. Torsion less than 15 degrees is internal tibial torsion; torsion greater than 30 degrees is external tibial torsion. This torsion is within the bone and cannot be changed by twisting the knee. Tibial torsion and femoral torsion can occur in any combination. Internal tibial torsion will either aggravate in-toeing if the child has anteverted hips or improve foot position if the child has

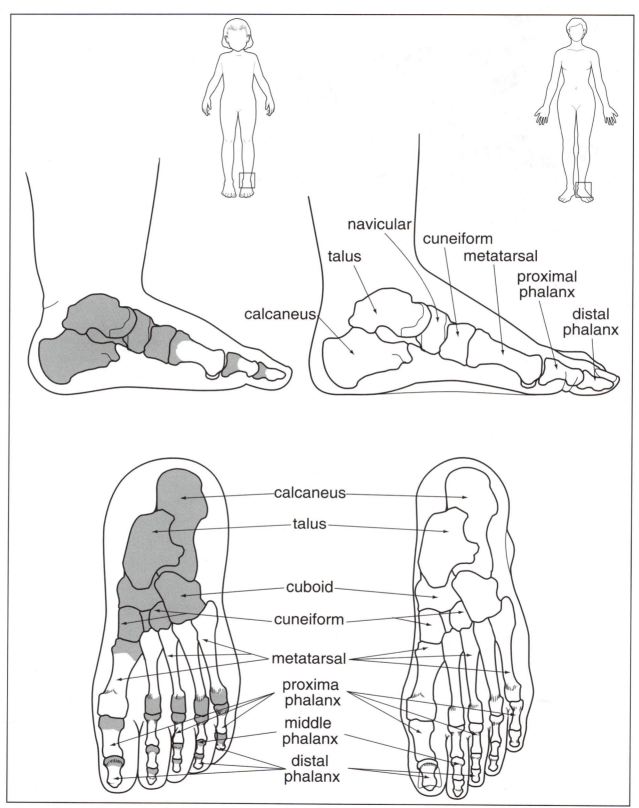

Figure 6.1. Ankle–Foot Skeletal System

retroverted hips. Conversely, external tibial torsion will aggravate out-toeing if the child has retroverted hips or improve foot position if the child has anteverted hips. In active children, these normally occurring torsions disappear by age 8 or 9. The torsions themselves do not prevent functional motion, especially ambulation.

The axis of motion determines the direction in which range of motion should occur. If a child has internal tibial torsion, the axis for range of motion is more horizontal than with external tibial torsion. If the axis is not considered, compression of one side of the joint while gapping the other side occurs during range-of-motion and weight-shifting activities in standing. Joint response to compression is defined as excitation of the joint receptors and subsequent contraction of the surrounding musculature. This normal protective contraction can be incorrectly interpreted as a spastic response.

To ensure range of motion occurs in the correct plane, locate the subtalor joint. Place it in close-packed position (supination). Then distract the posterior aspect of the calcaneus while compressing the distal aspect of the calcaneus. The force is applied perpendicular to the axis, and not distal to the transverse tarsal joint. If full passive range of motion of the talocrural joint (with subtalor joint close-packed) is unavailable, nothing can be said about muscle flexibility until this joint is free to move in this position.

Range of motion measurements are difficult in the ankle-foot complex because of the variety of planes involved, the angles of the bones, and the number of joints that contribute to a similarly named motion. Esch's technique for measuring ankle range of motion places one arm of the goniometer along the fibula while the other arm lines up with the fifth metatarsal (Esch and Lepley 1971). This method of measurement crosses the talocrural and the transverse tarsal joints; therefore, either joint could contribute to the measured motion. Because the foot in the child with cerebral palsy is frequently malaligned and overstretched in some joints and tight in others, do not assume that the motion measured according to Esch's method only records talocrural joint motion. In fact, a child with a rocker bottom foot (dorsiflexion of the transverse tarsal joint with plantarflexion of the talocrural joint) will show a dorsiflexion measurement using Esch's method. A more accurate reading can be obtained by measuring each joint individually. In this case, align one arm of the goniometer with the fibula and the other arm with the calcaneus to measure talocrural joint motion. To measure transverse tarsal dorsiflexion, align one arm of the goniometer with the calcaneus and the other with the cuboid and fifth metatarsal.

Among the few who have studied range of motion in the foot, Hensinger and Jone (1982) and Hoffer (1980) have studied range of motion in the newborn's foot; Giannestras (1973) and Jordan et al. (1983) have studied range of motion in the older child's foot; and McCrea (1985) and Tax (1985) have studied range of motion in both. These authors found that total flexion decreased from 70 degrees in the newborn to 45 to 50 degrees in the 6-month-old to 25 to 45 degrees in the 1-year-old. Conversely, extension gained range of motion, from 115 to 130 degrees in the neonate to 145 to 150 degrees in the 1-year-old. Pronation and supination range of motion appeared stable over time, though there is twice as much supination as pronation (Milgrom et al. 1985).

Ligamentous System

When examining the foot and ankle complex, it is critical to assess position and movement on a joint-by-joint basis before correcting.

The three joints of the foot that are primarily responsible for mobility and stability functions are composed of interlocking bones, with each bone participating in more than one joint. The talus is particularly important because it participates in all three joints.

Talocrural Joint

The talocrural joint is composed of the talus, tibia, and fibula. The ligaments are the crural tibiofibular interosseous ligament, anterior and posterior tibiofibular ligaments for the inferior tibiofibular joints, and the medial and lateral collateral ligaments of the ankle, and the deltoid. Motion available includes dorsiflexion and plantarflexion. Capsular patterns of restriction limit both plantar- and dorsiflexion.

The talocrural joint is supported by two additional joints: the superior and inferior tibiofibular joints (see Figure 5.1, page 50). The superior and inferior tibiofibular joints are synovial joints and do move during ankle dorsiflexion, especially at the end of the range. How the joint moves is debatable (laterally, superiorly, or rotary); however, movement of the fibula allows the wide anterior aspect of the talus to move into close-pack position in the mortise during terminal dorsiflexion.

Close-packed position of the talocrural joint is approximately 5 degrees of dorsiflexion. This is the position of the ankle during single limb stance during gait when joint stability is an asset.

Subtalor Joint

The subtalor joint is composed of the talus and calcaneus (Figure 6.2). It is supported by the medial and lateral collateral ligaments of the ankle, the interosseous talocalcaneal ligament, and the posterior and lateral talocalcaneal ligaments. The joint is close-packed in a position of slight supination. The capsular pattern of restriction produces a greater limitation to inversion than to eversion. This is the pattern usually seen in children with cerebral palsy.

Motion of the subtalor joint is triplanar. The triplanar motion is both supination and pronation. Supination is foot adduction around a vertical axis, inversion around a sagittal axis, and plantarflexion of the talus on the calcaneus around a coronal axis. Pronation is foot abduction around a vertical axis, eversion around a sagittal axis, and dorsiflexion of the talus on the calcaneus around a coronal axis. Note that the foot can be supinated and dorsiflexed, though supination of the subtalor joint requires plantarflexion between the calcaneus and the talus. This dorsiflexion occurs between the talus and the mortise while the talus is plantarflexed in relation to the calcaneus, allowing supination of the subtalor joint.

The axis of the joint is triplanar but more sagittal then coronal or vertical. Therefore, this joint allows more of the inversion component than the adduction and plantarflexion components of supination. This is in contrast to the motion allowed at the midtarsal joint.

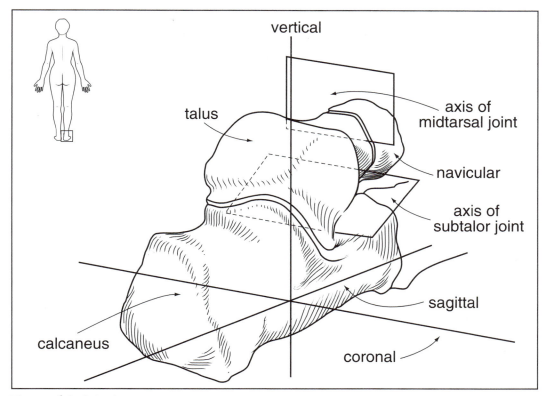

Figure 6.2. Subtalor Joint

Midtarsal Joint

This joint is composed of the talus, calcaneus, cuboid, and navicular. Ligaments are the bifurcate ligament (lateral band), dorsal and plantar calcaneocuboid, and long plantar ligaments, as well as the supports to the subtalor joint.

The motion available at this joint, supination and pronation, is also triplanar. Close-packed position is also slight supination.

In contrast to the subtalor joint, the axis of this joint is more vertical and coronal. This joint therefore allows more of the adduction and plantarflexion components of supination than the inversion component. This is particularly relevant to children with cerebral palsy, as they often have twisted feet. In other words, the "pronated" foot commonly seen in the child with spastic diplegic cerebral palsy is often a combination of subtalor eversion, transverse tarsal inversion, and transverse tarsal abduction. The joints are not pronated or supinated around their correct axes but twisted, with some of the component motions contributing more to the malalignment than others.

Assessing Ligament Flexibility

Table 6.1 lists techniques to assess ankle and foot ligament flexibility. To perform these techniques at the talocrural joint, stabilize the tibia and fibula at the malleoli with one hand and place the web space of the other hand over the talus located in between the malleoli (Figure 6.3). Push the talus posteriorly for more dorsiflexion; pull the talus anteriorly for more plantarflexion. To perform the techniques at the subtalor joint, one hand stabilizes the tibia, fibula, and talus while the other hand moves the calcaneus at the subtalor joint (Figure 6.4). The calcaneus can be moved along a triplanar, sagittal, coronal, or vertical axis. Mobilization or joint play assessment of the transverse tarsal joint is similar to the technique at the subtalor joint, except the hand placement is different (Figure 6.5). Stabilize the calcaneus with one hand and move the navicular and cuboid with the other hand to assess the transverse tarsal joint. The four planes of movement for this joint are the same as for the subtalor joint.

Table 6.1
Techniques to Assess Ankle-Foot Ligament Flexibility

Range	Technique	Hand Position	Force Direction
Talocrural: Dorsiflex	A–P glide	Stabilize the tibia and fibula; mobilize the talus.	Talus moves posteriorly.
Plantar	P–A glide	Stabilize the tibia and fibula; mobilize the talus.	Talus moves anteriorly.
Subtalor:			
	Supination	Stabilize the talus and mobilize the calcaneus.	Calcaneus in triplanar direction.
	Dorsiflexion	Stabilize the talus and mobilize the calcaneus.	Calcaneus around a coronal axis.
	Plantarflexion	Stabilize the talus and mobilize the calcaneus.	Calcaneus around a coronal axis.
	Abduction	Stabilize the talus and mobilize the calcaneus.	Calcaneus around a vertical axis.
	Adduction	Stabilize the talus and mobilize the calcaneus.	Calcaneus around a vertical axis.
	Inversion	Stabilize the talus and mobilize the calcaneus.	Calcaneus around a sagittal axis.
	Eversion	Stabilize the talus and mobilize the calcaneus.	Calcaneus around a sagittal axis.
Midtarsal:			
	Supination	Stabilize the talus and calcaneus and mobilize the navicular and cuboid.	Calcaneus in triplanar direction.
	Dorsiflexion	Stabilize the talus and calcaneus and mobilize the navicular and cuboid.	Calcaneus around a coronal axis.
	Plantarflexion	Stabilize the talus and calcaneus and mobilize the navicular and cuboid.	Calcaneus around a coronal axis.
	Abduction	Stabilize the talus and calcaneus and mobilize the navicular and cuboid.	Calcaneus around a vertical axis.
	Adduction	Stabilize the talus and calcaneus and mobilize the navicular and cuboid.	Calcaneus around a vertical axis.
	Inversion	Stabilize the talus and calcaneus and mobilize the navicular and cuboid.	Calcaneus around a sagittal axis.
	Eversion	Stabilize the talus and calcaneus and mobilize the navicular and cuboid.	Calcaneus around a sagittal axis.
Great toe:			
	Dorsiflexion	Stabilize the metatarsal and mobilize the phalanx.	Phalanx moves dorsally.

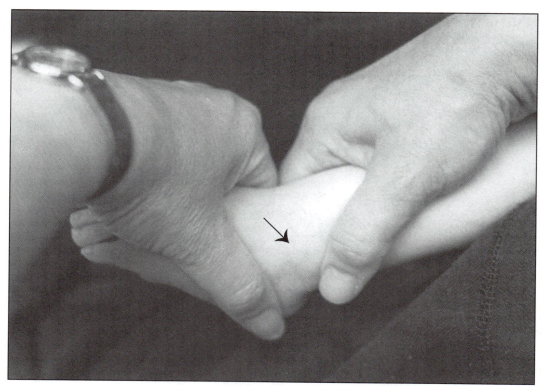

Figure 6.3. Anterior and Posterior Glides

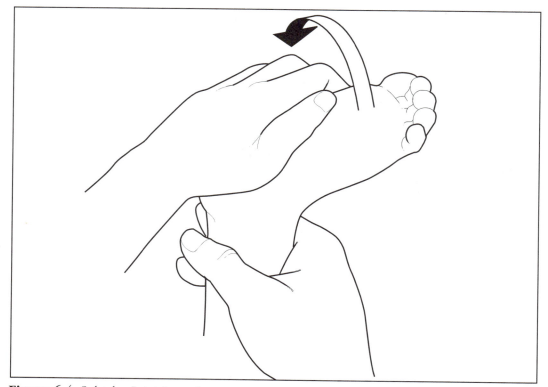

Figure 6.4. Subtalor Joint Inversion

The joints of the ankle/foot complex function as a group to achieve mobility and stability. The foot is mobile in initial weightbearing to absorb the rotary stress placed upon it, then stable at midstance and finally a rigid lever at push-off. At initial contact, the calcaneus becomes pronated at the subtalor joint. This is an open-packed position, allowing the foot at the midtarsal joint to conform to the ground. At midstance, the foot must be a stable base of support for single limb stance. The stable base of support occurs as the close-pack position of the subtalor joint leads to close-pack position of the midtarsal joint. What results is a very stable foot and a rigid lever for push-off.

The shift of body weight causes the joints to shift from pronation to supination. Notice that in initial contact, body weight is medial to the axis of the joint, and the joint moves into pronation. As the body weight shifts laterally in single limb stance, weight shifts lateral to the joint axis, resulting in supination of the foot.

This shift in weightbearing shifts the axis, resulting in changes in muscular activity. In normal motion the gastrocsoleous, anterior tibialis, and the posterior tibialis act as supinators, and the peroneals act as pronators. But if the axis of the subtalor joint is significantly displaced medially (as in severe pronation), the anterior tibialis, posterior tibialis, and gastrocsoleous all pull lateral to the displaced axis, producing pronation. Many children with cerebral palsy have active anterior tibialis muscles, but when these contract, the forefoot abducts and pronates. The forefoot can only do this if the subtalor joint axis is lateral to the anterior tibialis tendon. Joints must be realigned before strengthening or stretching of muscles will have the desired effect on functional movement (Figure 6.6).

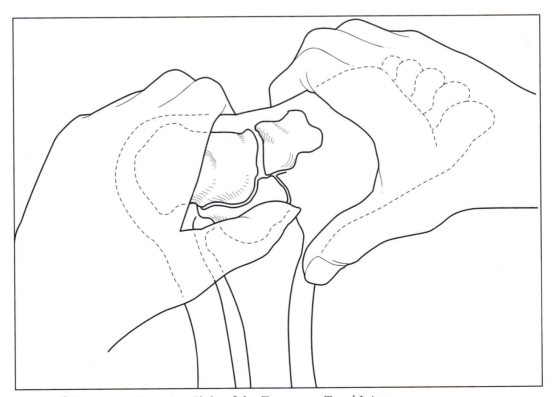

Figure 6.5. Anterior-Posterior Glide of the Transverse Tarsal Joint

Muscular System

Carefully assess the flexibility, strength, and endurance of the musculature in light of joint range of motion. Rule out substitutions because it is easy to confuse joint limitation, weakness, and tightness. This is clearly demonstrated in testing muscle flexibility at the talocrural joint. The common test of flexibility for the ankle involves dorsiflexing the ankle with the knee flexed and then extending the knee to differentiate between the flexibility of the gastrocnemius and the soleus. However, this test is not accurate (Perry et al. 1974). Children with cerebral palsy often have a limitation to full passive range of motion at the ankle, even with the knee flexed. No inferences can be made regarding muscle flexibility until the joint play is assessed and replaced if necessary. Once full ankle joint range of motion is available with the knee flexed, then muscle flexibility can be assessed by extending the knee. It is normal for the gastrocsoleous muscle group to decrease the total available range of motion at the ankle with the knee extended (as opposed to when the knee is flexed).

Gait does not require the total range of 25 to 30 degrees of dorsiflexion at the ankle and full muscle flexibility with the knee extended. In fact, some children with cerebral palsy attain that amount of range after heel cord surgery and still ambulate with a very inefficient crouch gait. This inefficiency is frequently related to weakness in the gastrocsoleus.

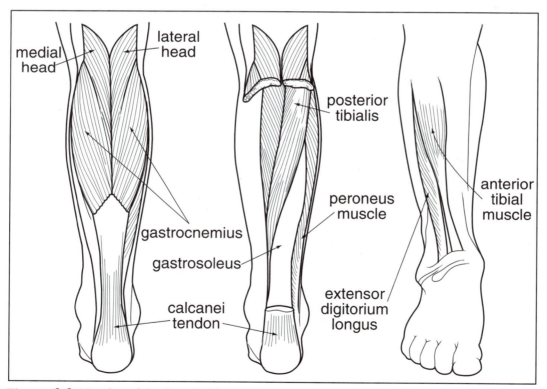

Figure 6.6. Muscles of the Foot/Ankle

Table 6.2
Ankle-Foot Muscle Flexibility Testing for Children with Cerebral Palsy

Muscle Group	Testing Techniques	Substitutions
Dorsiflexors	Stabilize the mortise and plantarflex.	Plantarflexion in eversion at the subtalor/transverse tarsal joint
Plantarflexors	Stabilize the mortise and dorsiflex with supination.	Dorsiflex occurs only in eversion with the range coming from the subtalor or transverse tarsal joints.
Invertors	Stabilize the mortise and evert subtalor joint.	Inversion occurs only with plantarflexion.
Evertors	Stabilize the mortise and invert subtalor joint.	Eversion occurs only to neutral.
Great toe flexor	Stabilize the mortise, subtalor, and transverse tarsal joints; extend the great toe.	Extension only to neutral.

Muscle Strength

Muscle strength at the foot and ankle must be considered from non-weightbearing and weightbearing perspectives. In non-weightbearing, the ankle musculature moves against the resistance of the foot and possibly a shoe. In weightbearing, the ankle muscles move the body's weight against the fixed foot. Non-weightbearing testing will not address strength needs for functional weightbearing.

Many children with cerebral palsy do not have the concentric/eccentric strength to wiggle the foot, even in non-weightbearing. Some infants with cerebral palsy do not even wiggle their feet while lying supine or in response to tickling, while other children with cerebral palsy show only isometric strength. These children often walk on their toes, or on the balls of their feet, and seldom stand flat-footed before going up on their toes with a concentric contraction. Frequently, they plantarflex the foot before standing on it and maintain the contraction isometrically while standing. Other children have the necessary strength, but only when the joint axes are aligned. These children may need bracing or surgery to maintain the alignment for proper muscle functioning.

Muscle strength critical to efficient ambulation includes at least good strength concentrically and eccentrically in the gastrocsoleus group. Whereas many children with cerebral palsy stand with isometric contractions of the gastrocsoleus group, very few can use concentric and eccentric contractions to go up and down on their toes. Even fewer can use eccentric and concentric contractions of the gastrocsoleus unilaterally as is necessary for push-off in gait. Heel cord lengthenings can have a devastating effect on strength, push-off, and efficiency in gait.

Table 6.3
Proposed Strength Criteria for Ankle-Foot Musculature

Strength Criteria	Dorsiflex	Plantarflex
Poor (Movement with gravity eliminated.)	Full range in sidelying	Full range in sidelying
Fair (Movement against gravity.)	Full range in supine	Full range in supine
Good (Movement against gravity and some resistance.)	Full range with some resistance, i.e., shoes	Full range with some resistance, i.e., shoes
Normal (Age-appropriate resistance.)	Full range with age-appropriate resistance	N.A.
At 3 months	Wiggles feet antigravity.	Wiggles feet antigravity.
At 6 months	N.A.	N.A.
At 9 months	Pulls to stand over foot.	Pulls to stand over foot.
At 12 months	Weight shifts at ankle.	Weights shifts at ankle.
At 18 months	Squats.	Squats.
At 24 months	Jumps.	Jumps.
At 36 months	Heel-toe appears in gait.	Heel-toe appears in gait.

N.A. Not available

Muscle Endurance

Although quality of movement has its place in therapy, so does quantity. Eventually, arriving at a destination is more important than the gait used. This is very apparent in the child who has just spent time in therapy to ambulate with heel strike 5 or 10 feet, but who then rushes out of therapy on her toes to get to the next class.

This is because children with cerebral palsy can only contract and relax ankle musculature a fraction of the frequency required for normal gait (i.e., 70 to 80 times per minute per foot). This is due to either neurologic damage or poor muscular endurance. Muscular endurance as a contributing factor is amenable to training programs, but the neurological damage may limit the extent of improvement in speed of rapid alternating movements.

Treatment Planning

In the patient with neurological damage, the foot is frequently distorted. It may be pronated, supinated, plantarflexed, and twisted. Common terminology frequently confuses the management of the foot. Terms used to describe the foot are global (i.e., "pronated foot"). However, because each joint of the foot contributes to the deformity, each must be individually assessed and managed. The foot deformities commonly seen in children with cerebral palsy are grouped into four very broad categories: the plantarflexed foot, the rocker bottom foot, the hemiplegic foot, and the diplegic foot. Each broad category is only an example of the kind of existing deformities. Each child's foot can be any combination of correct and incorrect alignment. This discussion is a guide to some of the multiple problems a globally described foot may exhibit.

The Plantarflexed Foot

Plantarflexion occurs with significant range at two joints in the foot. Classically, the talocrural articulation is assessed and managed when a foot is described as plantarflexed. Frequently, additional plantarflexion occurs at the midtarsal joint. Flexibility for dorsiflexion at the midtarsal joint is critical for the foot to splay to accept body weight and for normal supination and pronation for weight shift. Because the axis of the subtalor joint has very little coronal orientation, there is very little plantarflexion available at the subtalor joint.

To assess the range from each joint, modify classic landmarks for range of motion. To assess the range from the talocrural joint, place one arm of the goniometer on the fibula and the other arm on the calcaneus.

To measure plantarflexion at the midtarsal joint, place one arm of the goniometer on the calcaneus and the other arm on the fifth metatarsal. Plantarflexion here may mimic plantarflexion at the talocrural joint. This is usually a limitation of joint play as the flexibility of the gastrocsoleous does not affect this joint position. If the foot is plantarflexed only at the talocrural joint, mobilization may be indicated between the talus and tibia-fibula. However, if plantarflexion is found at the midtarsal joint, mobilization may be indicated, but this time between the talus-calcaneus and cuboid navicular.

Table 6.4
Evaluation and Treatment Considerations in the "Plantarflexed Foot"

System	Findings	Treatment Options
Skeletal	Vertical talus	Surgery
Ligamentous	Talocrural joint limit	Mobilize talocrural joint.
	Transverse tarsal joint limit	Mobilize transverse tarsal.
Muscular	Tight gastrocsoleous	Stretch or surgery
	Tight toe flexor and/or foot intrinsics	Stretch the appropriate muscles.
	Weak anterior tibialis	Strengthen muscle.
Neurological	Peripheral neuropathy subsequent to casting	Stabilize joints until nerve regeneration.
	Abnormal reflexes, stiffness	Classic neurological techniques

The Rocker Bottom Foot

The rocker bottom foot occurs when the talus is plantarflexed relative to the tibia and fibula at the same time that the midtarsal joint is dorsiflexed. This can occur whenever weight-bearing is forced on a foot with insufficient ankle joint mobility, or when the foot and ankle are forced into a splint set at 90 degrees when the ankle joint has less than 90 degrees of range available.

Measurement techniques for these joints have already been described. Evaluation and treatment consideration are the same as the "plantarflexed foot" and the "hemiplegic foot."

The Hemiplegic Foot

The foot frequently seen in children with hemiplegia is often described as supinated. This term is misleading because the ankle cannot be supinated. It is the subtalor joint that can be supinated or pronated; the midtarsal joint, on the other hand, is frequently adducted. Again, each joint must be treated individually. That is, if the ankle is plantarflexed, the subtalor joint is pronated, and the midtarsal joint is adducted, the "supinated" foot cannot be managed by pronating it. Instead, the ankle must have mobility for dorsiflexion, the subtalor joint must be supinated, and the midtarsal joint must be abducted.

To assess the subtalor joint position, determine the subtalor joint's neutral position. When the talus is balanced between the malleoli (neutral), a line bisecting the calcaneus and a line perpendicular to the support should form an angle. In the child 3 years old or younger, this angle is 3 to 5 degrees medial due to the valgus position of the calcaneus at this age. In the child over the age of 5, this angle is 3 to 5 degrees lateral due to the varus position of the calcaneus at this age. Supination and pronation are the mobility from this neutral position. Only careful assessment of the mechanical alignment within the age norms can reveal malalignment in supination or pronation at this joint. In the "hemiplegic foot," the subtalor joint may be in either position.

The midtarsal joint is assessed after the subtalor joint is aligned. The axis of the foot is sagittal along the second ray. This axis bisects the tibia in the aligned joint. Malalignment of the midtarsal joint is evident when a line parallel to the second ray does not bisect the tibia, clearly demonstrating the joint to be adducted. Treatment of the foot requires realignment of each joint based on its relative position. This principle applies equally to treatment as well as orthotic management.

Table 6.5
Evaluation and Treatment Considerations in the "Hemiplegic Foot"

System	Findings	Treatment Options
Skeletal	Bone deformity	Surgery or bracing
Ligamentous	Hypermobility or hypomobility in the talocrural, subtalor, or transverse tarsal joints	Brace or surgically fix the laxity; mobilize the hypomobility.
Muscular	Limited flexibility	Stretch muscles until limiting range of motion if joint mobility is present.
	Weakness	Strengthen muscles if alignment of the joints can be maintained.

The Diplegic Foot

The foot frequently seen in the child with spastic diplegia is often described as pronated. As with the "hemiplegic foot," each joint must be individually assessed and treated. Often the child with spastic diplegia has a plantarflexed talocrural joint, pronated subtalor joint, and abducted and inverted midtarsal joint. That is why simply supinating the foot does not produce normal alignment. These assessment and treatment options utilize the same principles as those described for the "hemiplegic" foot.

These descriptions of common malalignments are examples of frequently seen deformities. Any combination of malalignments may occur. Only individual assessment and problem solving can address the problems of a specific patient. This is critical not only for alignment for exercise, but also for alignment in splinting.

For example, the diplegic foot often has talocrural plantarflexion, subtalor eversion, and midtarsal inversion and abduction. The talocrural joint is close-packed (stable) at 5 degrees of dorsiflexion. When the child is in an ankle-foot orthosis set at neutral, the joints are in an inherently unstable position. Hence the ankle-foot orthosis, trying to provide stability, may actually place the ankle in an unstable position. The midtarsal joint inversion becomes obvious when the subtalor joint is properly aligned. To address this alignment problem, the ankle-foot orthosis would need to hold the subtalor joint in neutral and evert the midtarsal joint. Unfortunately, it is common for the ankle-foot orthosis to allow the subtalor joint to evert and apply inversion pressure under the midtarsal joint. Once again, each joint of the foot must be assessed and corrected individually.

Summary

The foot provides mobility and stability through the interaction of the talocrural, subtalor, and midtarsal joints. Global descriptions of malalignment in the feet of children with cerebral palsy frequently mask the twisted nature of the actual malalignments.

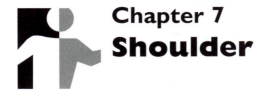

Chapter 7
Shoulder

The shoulder girdle is a complex of the sternoclavicular, acromioclavicular, scapulothoracic, and glenohumoral joints.

Skeletal System

Bones involved in the shoulder girdle are the clavicle, scapula, sternum, and humerus (Figure 7.1); all have very shallow articulations and are highly dependent upon their ligamentous integrity for support.

Normal range of motion at the shoulder in children has not been well studied. However, the question of whether joint motion in the cardinal plane and in the plane of the scapula are the same has been addressed. In the 3-year-old, values for abduction of the glenohumoral joint in the frontal plane are 90 to 135 degrees, as opposed to values for abduction in the plane of the scapula of 107 to 115 degrees (Doody and Waterland 1970; Freedman and Munroe 1966). Neither of these values is anywhere near the often quoted norm of almost 170 degrees of abduction in the adult. Use caution when applying passive range to the infant.

Ligamentous System

Sternoclavicular Joint

The sternoclavicular joint is composed of the sternum and the clavicle. The ligaments are the anterior and posterior sternoclavicular ligaments and the costoclavicular and interclavicular ligaments. Figure 7.2 shows the anatomical relationship in the infant.

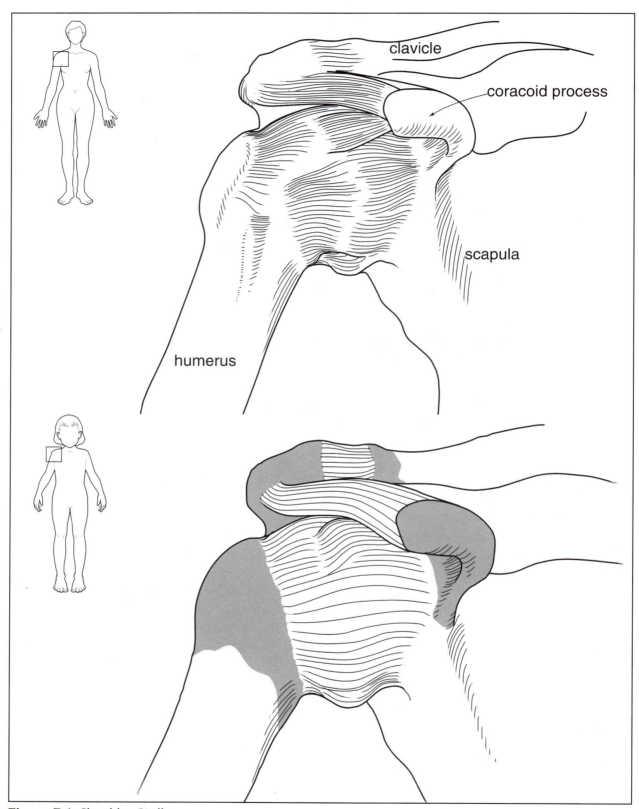

Figure 7.1. Shoulder Girdle

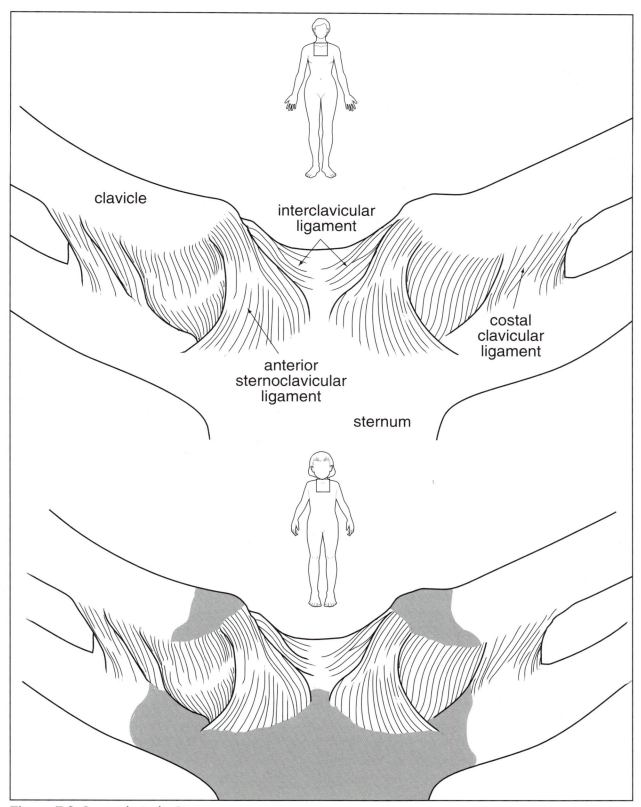

clavicle

interclavicular
ligament

costal
clavicular
ligament

anterior
sternoclavicular
ligament

sternum

Figure 7.2. Sternoclavicular Ligaments

The capsular pattern of ligamentous tightness is a limitation of elevation and protraction of the distal end of the clavicle relative to the proximal end. Even though many children with cerebral palsy appear to have elevated and protracted shoulders, the distal end of the clavicle is not elevated or protracted relative to the proximal end. This apparent paradox is explained by the alignment of the clavicle relative to the sternum when the spine is kyphosed. Children with cerebral palsy appear to have elevated and protracted shoulders when the spine is kyphosed. Once the spine is extended, the clavicle is neutral relative to the sternum and the joint has little or no elevation and protraction—and both are critical for reach.

The sternoclavicular joint is the only bone connection between the upper extremity and the trunk. The motions available are clavicular elevation/depression, protraction/retraction, and rotation. The costoclavicular ligament provides the axis of motion for elevation and depression, as well as protraction and retraction. This ligament is located outside of the joint and results in a see-saw motion. Rotation occurs along the long axis and requires additional movement at the acromioclavicular joint.

Acromioclavicular Joint

The acromioclavicular joint is composed of the acromion of the scapula and the clavicle. The ligaments are the superior and inferior acromioclavicular and the coracoclavicular ligaments.

Close-packed position of the joint occurs during upward rotation and protraction of the scapula, as in reaching. In the adult, this joint contributes to shoulder elevation after 60 degrees and stops contributing motion between 90 and 120 degrees of elevation (Kessler and Hertling 1983). Because this joint is a fibrocartilagenous union until almost 2 years of age (Cailliet 1966), it is theoretically unable to contribute to the scapulohumeral rhythm in the child as it does in the adult. This may explain the more limited range of motion norms identified for children by Freedman and Munroe (1966) and Doody and Waterland (1970). It is possible then that total range of motion in the infant and child is markedly different and more limited than in the adult. Observation of normal infants does suggest that they do not show 170 degrees of shoulder abduction or flexion.

This joint maintains the relationship between the clavicle and the scapula in the early stages of elevation and allows additional range of scapular rotation in the latter stages of elevation. Motions available are scapular rotation, winging, and tipping. Scapular rotation occurs in an upward/downward direction during upper extremity elevation at the same time that the scapula glides over the thorax. Winging occurs when the vertebral border of the scapula rides perpendicular to the thorax. Tipping is the normal alignment of the flat scapula as it rides forward over the round thorax, as occurs in kyphosis. Tipping is frequently seen in children with cerebral palsy; winging is not.

Scapulothoracic Joint

The scapulothoracic joint is not a synovial joint but a fascial plane between the thoracic and scapular muscles. No ligaments support the relationship and therefore no capsular pattern of restriction exists. It is atmospheric pressure that is thought to hold the scapula to the thorax (Steindler 1973). This joint moves as a result of motion at the sternoclavicular and acromioclavicular joints. Consequently, limitations there will limit scapulothoracic motion. Many approaches to management of motor disorders in children with cerebral palsy have focused on the scapula. The anatomy suggests that focus needs to shift to mobility at the sterno- and acromioclavicular joints.

The purpose of the joint is to orient the glenoid fossa. Motions available are scapular elevation/depression, abduction/adduction, and upward/downward rotation. Scapular elevation and depression occur in conjunction with sternoclavicular elevation and depression. Scapular abduction and adduction are associated with clavicular protraction and retraction. Scapular upward and downward rotation is associated with acromioclavicular joint motion.

Glenohumoral Joint

The glenohumoral joint is composed of the scapula and humerus. It is supported by the coracohumeral and glenohumeral ligaments. Figure 7.1 illustrates the anatomical relationships in the infant. The coracohumeral ligament passively supports the humerus in the joint. Close-packed position of this joint is abduction, external rotation, and flexion. The capsular pattern of restriction includes maximum limitation to external rotation, considerable limitation to abduction, and relatively free flexion and internal rotation. Children with cerebral palsy frequently have a significant limitation to external rotation and abduction, with relatively free internal rotation and flexion.

Motions available at the joint are flexion/extension, abduction/adduction, and internal/external rotation. Any limitation to movement at the other three joints of the shoulder girdle can put undue stress on the support structures of the glenohumoral joint, which may result in laxity of part of the glenohumoral joint. Any excess flexibility of these ligaments can cause a subluxation; it is no coincidence that some children with cerebral palsy are quite adept at subluxing the glenohumoral joint. Perhaps the problem is not the laxity at the glenohumoral joint but the limitation at the sternoclavicular and acromioclavicular joints.

Table 7.1 lists techniques to assess shoulder girdle ligaments. Figure 7.3 illustrates the hand positions for the technique at the sternoclavicular joint. To mobilize the sternoclavicular joint, stabilize the trunk at the sternum, grasp the clavicle, and move it in the requisite direction. Because techniques for the acromioclavicular joint are usually painful, do not use them on children. The range at this joint can be achieved by having the child in prone push backwards in crawling or push back into sitting with the aim between 60 and 90 degrees of elevation. Myofascial techniques are appropriate at the scapulothoracic joint, but mobilization of the glenohumoral joint is generally unnecessary.

Table 7.1
Techniques to Assess Shoulder Ligament Flexibility

Range	Technique	Hand Position	Force Direction
S–C elevation	Inferior glide	Stabilize the sternum and mobilize the clavicle.	Distal end of the clavicle elevates.
S–C protraction	Posterior glide	Stabilize the sternum and mobilize the clavicle.	Distal end of clavicle protracts.
A–C mobility	Compression	Stabilize the clavicle and scapula; push the two together.	Clavicle opens posteriorly, scapula moves anteriorly.
Glenohumeral flexion	Inferior glide	Stabilize the scapula and mobilize the humerus.	Humerus moves inferiorly.
Glenohumeral abduction	Inferior glide	Stabilize the scapula and mobilize the humerus.	Humerus moves inferiorly.
Glenohumeral external rotation	P–A glide	Stabilize the scapula and mobilize the humerus.	Humerus moves anteriorly.

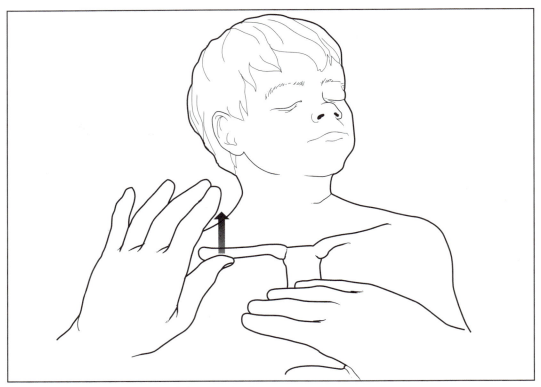

Figure 7.3. Inferior Glide Mobilization Technique

Scapulohumoral Rhythm

Each joint acts in a pattern of scapulohumoral rhythm. This rhythm is a 2:1 relationship between the scapula and the humerus during movement. That is, for every 2 degrees that the humerus moves, the scapula moves 1 degree. This ratio, however, is variable within the range. The initial third of the range of motion is primarily glenohumoral. This is consistent with the acromioclavicular joint's role of maintaining the relationship between the scapula and clavicle in the initial stages of elevation. During the middle third of the range of abduction or flexion, the sternoclavicular and acromioclavicular joints contribute range along with the humerus. The sternoclavicular joint contributes the most range (30 degrees) and does so in the early phase of this stage. The acromioclavicular joint contributes range from approximately 90 degrees to 120 degrees by allowing rotation through the longitudinal axis of the clavicle. Again, this is consistent with the acromioclavicular joint's purpose, which is to allow additional range of scapular rotation in a later stage of shoulder elevation. The humerus contributes only a few degrees in the middle third of the total range. The final third of the range of motion is contributed primarily by the humerus on the scapula.

It is the middle third of the range of motion where children with cerebral palsy tend to have range limitation, suggesting compromised flexibility of the sternoclavicular and acromioclavicular joints. However, before application of any shoulder assessment or treatment, identification of the actual alignment is critical. For example, the child who sacral-sits will apparently have elevated and protracted shoulders. But once the pelvis is aligned over the femurs, the actual position of the joints can be ascertained. Frequently, the shoulder girdle is not elevated and protracted; but immobility exists in the sternoclavicular and acromioclavicular joints along with increased mobility in the glenohumeral joint. If the assessment's theoretical perspective assumes the shoulder girdle is elevated and protracted, then the treatment will depress and retract the girdle. If the shoulder girdle is simply stuck, then elevate and protract the sternoclavicular joint as is necessary for the normal mechanics in reaching.

Muscular System

Decreased flexibility in the shoulder is frequently credited as the cause of the apparently protracted and elevated shoulder girdle in children with cerebral palsy. As discussed above, joint limitations and special malalignments also contribute to the posture. The shoulder muscles, however, must be aligned on their base (the trunk) before their flexibility can be assessed. The kyphotic posture so commonly seen in children with these rounded shoulders must be addressed before assessment of shoulder muscle flexibility.

Table 7.2 lists techniques to assess muscular flexibility once the spine is aligned.

Table 7.2
Shoulder Flexibility Testing for Children with Cerebral Palsy

Muscle Group	Testing Technique	Substitutions
Shoulder abductors	Scarf sign	Rolling or trunk rotation
Shoulder flexors	Stabilize scapula, extend elbow and shoulder.	Shift center of gravity back and flex trunk.
Shoulder extensors	Stabilize scapula, flex elbow and shoulder.	Flex trunk.
Shoulder external rotators	Stabilize scapula; internal rotation dependent on humerus.	Turning the trunk.
Shoulder internal rotators	Stabilize scapula; external rotation dependent on humerus.	Flex trunk.

The muscles of elevation are the deltoid, supraspinatous, infraspinatus, teres minor, subscapularis, trapezius serratus anterior, and rhomboids. The muscles of depression are the latissimus dorsi, pectorals, teres major, and rhomboids. These muscles are frequently overly active in the child with cerebral palsy who sacral-sits or ambulates with a supportive device. Sacral-sitting shifts the center of gravity behind the pelvis and therefore puts the shoulder muscles in the unusual role of trunk supporter against gravity. Children either fall backward or must use muscles to shift parts of the body forward over the base of support, because they cannot shift the center of gravity forward even though the abdominals and hip flexors support the trunk. Instead, the spine rounds and the arms come forward as the children try to hold onto their knees or the support surface. If the shoulder muscles are supporting the body against gravity, it is very difficult to raise the arm to reach. Furthermore, because the weight of the arm is counterbalancing the center of gravity, raising the arm tends to throw children backward. Joint range, ligamentous flexibility, and muscular strength cannot be accurately assessed until the center of gravity is placed forward over the femurs.

Because the internal and external rotators are also abductors/adductors or flexors/extensors of the shoulders, and children do not have the motor control to test these muscles in isolation, strength in these actions is inferred from strength in the muscle's other actions.

Table 7.3 lists suggested criteria for muscle strength in children.

Table 7.3
Proposed Strength Criteria for Shoulder Muscles

Strength Criteria	Flexors	Extensors	Abductors	Adductors	External Rotation	Internal Rotation
Poor (Movement with gravity eliminated.)	Sidelying flexion.	Sidelying, extends arm from flexed position.	Prone or supine elevation on support.	Supported in sitting, arm comes to midline.	—	—
Fair (Movement against gravity.)	Sitting flexion.	Rocking in prone on hands, commando crawling.	Sitting abduction in plane of scapula.	Rocking in prone on hands, commando crawling.	Prone, arm dependent, externally rotated.	Supine swiping at toys, arms off of support onto stomach.
Good (Movement against gravity and some resistance.)	Sitting flexion with something in the hand, elbow straight.	Pushing body up against gravity, i.e., scooting.	Sitting abduction in plane of scapula with some resistance and extend elbow or toy in hand.	Pushing body up against gravity, i.e., scooting.	As with adductors, with some resistance.	As with adductors, with some resistance.
Normal (Age-appropriate resistance.)	Sitting flexion with age-appropriate items in hand, elbow straight.	Hoisting body on fixed arms.	Abduction in sitting in plane of scapula with age-appropriate resistance.	Hoisting body on fixed arms.	As with adduction, with age-appropriate resistance.	As with adduction, with age-appropriate resistance.
At 3 months	Thrusts arm in play through available range; prone pushups.	Partially elevates self by arms.	Thrusts arm in play through available range.	Partially elevates self by arms.	Swimming	Hands to midline
At 6 months	N.A.	Shifts weight on arms, pulls to sit.	Reaches in sitting.	Shifts weight on arms, pulls to sit.	Reaching for suspended ring	N.A.
At 9 months	N.A.	Raises self to standing with arms.	N.A.	Raises self to standing with arms.	N.A.	N.A.
At 12 months	N.A.	N.A.	N.A.	N.A.	N.A.	N.A.
At 18 months	Throws ball.	N.A.	Throws ball.	N.A.	N.A.	N.A.
At 24 months	Tosses a ring, begins feeding self with utensils.	N.A.	Tosses a ring.	N.A.	N.A.	N.A.
At 36 months	Throws heavy objects.	N.A.	N.A.	N.A.	Pitching toys	N.A.

N.A. Not available; unable to infer from standarized assessments.

Endurance in the shoulder musculature is needed for upper extremity functions such as dressing, and many children with cerebral palsy also need shoulder muscle endurance for ambulation. Crutches, canes, and walkers place increased stress on upper extremity musculature while decreasing the stress on the lower extremity musculature.

Treatment Planning

Elevated and Protracted Shoulders

Children with cerebral palsy are commonly described as having elevated and protracted shoulders. It is not surprising, then, that therapists frequently work on depression and retraction. The functional purpose of the shoulder, however, is to assist reach, placing the hand for function. Although reach usually requires some component of elevation and protraction, careful joint assessment of the child with cerebral palsy often reveals general immobility of the acromioclavicular and sternoclavicular joints, not necessarily limitation in any given direction. Once the mobility of the acromioclavicular and sternoclavicular joints is present, then strength and flexibility can be assessed. If joint range is available but the child does not raise the arm against gravity through the available range, weakness is a distinct possibility. When range and strength are present, then speed of movement, accuracy in placement, and endurance for an activity can be addressed.

Other joint systems affect placement of the shoulder girdle over the center of gravity. The spine must have extension available to place the shoulder girdle on its base to determine any malalignment problems. The hip joint requires full flexibility to allow the placement of the center of gravity over the base of support. Hamstrings must have sufficient strength to control the body weight forward with the added resistance of the elevated arm; however, hamstring flexibility is not usually a factor, since the knee is generally flexed in an upper extremity function as when tailor-sitting or when seated in a chair.

Table 7.4 lists common evaluation and treatment options.

Table 7.4
**Common Evaluation Results and Treatment Options
in Elevated or Protracted Shoulders**

System	Findings	Treatment Options
Skeletal		
Ligamentous	Decreased hip flexibility	Mobilization
	Decreased spine extension	Mobilization
	Decreased sternoclavicular, acromioclavicular, or glenohumeral flexibility	Mobilization
Muscular	Decreased strength in the hamstrings	Strengthen hamstrings at greater than 90 degrees flexion.
	Decreased back strength	Strengthen back extensors.
	Decreased shoulder musculature	Strengthen musculature.

Summary

The shoulder places the hand for function due to the coordinated action of four joints: the sternoclavicular, acromioclavicular, scapulothoracic, and glenohumeral joints. These joints coordinate their action in scapulohumoral rhythm. Limitation in movement in any one or two joints can produce excess mobility in another. In children with cerebral palsy, limited mobility of the sternoclavicular and acromioclavicular joints produces characteristic limitations to range, predictable motor problems and, often, hypermobility of the glenohumeral joint.

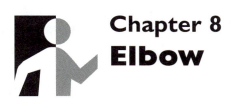

Chapter 8
Elbow

Skeletal System

Bones of the elbow are the humerus, ulna, and sometimes the radius (Figure 8.1). The elbow is supported by the superior and inferior radioulnar joints. The elbow and superior radioulnar joints are both contained within the elbow joint capsule, but they are distinct joints.

The articulation between the humerus and ulna allows flexion and extension of the elbow joint. The radius articulates with the humerus only in flexion of the joint. As the joint moves into extension, the radial head moves down and away from the humerus. If the two bones become unable to move away from each other, an apparent flexion contracture will be present. This may be part of the apparent elbow flexion contracture seen in children with cerebral palsy.

The radius articulates with the ulna at the superior and inferior radioulnar joints. These joints supinate and pronate the forearm.

Range of motion for flexion, extension, pronation, and supination has not been documented in infants and children; therefore caution against over-stretching must be stressed. The lack of range of motion research also holds obvious implications for future research.

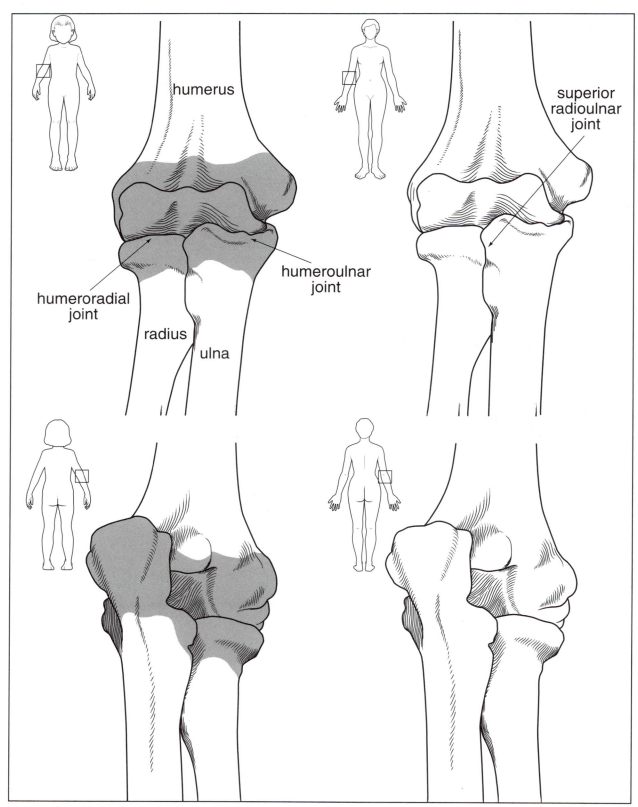

Figure 8.1. Elbow Skeletal System

Ligamentous System

The elbow joint is supported by the medial and lateral collateral ligaments. These ligaments, along with the bone shape, limit medial and lateral motion of the joint (Figure 8.2).

The annular ligament supports the radial head against the ulna at the superior radial ulnar joint (see Figure 8.2). This ligament limits motion of the radial head against the ulna to an almost pure spin. The motion available at this joint is supination and pronation, which occurs both at the superior and inferior radial ulnar joint. The quadrate ligament and the oblique cord support the superior radioulnar joints while the anterior and posterior radioulnar ligaments support the inferior radioulnar joint (see Figure 8.2). Involvement of the ligaments in the distal radioulnar joint seldom limits much motion but can be responsible for a pain at the end of the ranges of motion. Capsular restriction of the proximal joint, however, will almost completely limit supination; this may also be responsible for the radial head's inability to glide away from the humerus in elbow extension. Combining a limited mobility of the radial head upon both the humerus and ulna may explain the flexion pronation contracture in the arm of many children with cerebral palsy.

Table 8.1 lists techniques to assess ligamentous integrity of the joints. Techniques for flexion and extension are seldom used in children because of the potential for heterotopic ossificans. The technique for supination can be highly effective in the pronation and flexion contracture seen in many children with cerebral palsy. To perform the technique, stabilize the ulna and oscillate the radial head posteriorly (Figure 8.3). This technique is usually painful, so use caution.

Table 8.1
Techniques to Assess Elbow Ligament Flexibility

Range	Technique	Hand Position	Force Direction
Extension	—	Do not do with child.	—
Flexion	—	Do not do with child.	—
Supination	A–P glide	Stabilize the ulna and mobilize the radius.	Push the radial head posteriorly.
Pronation	P–A glide	Stabilize the ulna and mobilize the radius.	Push the radial head anteriorly.

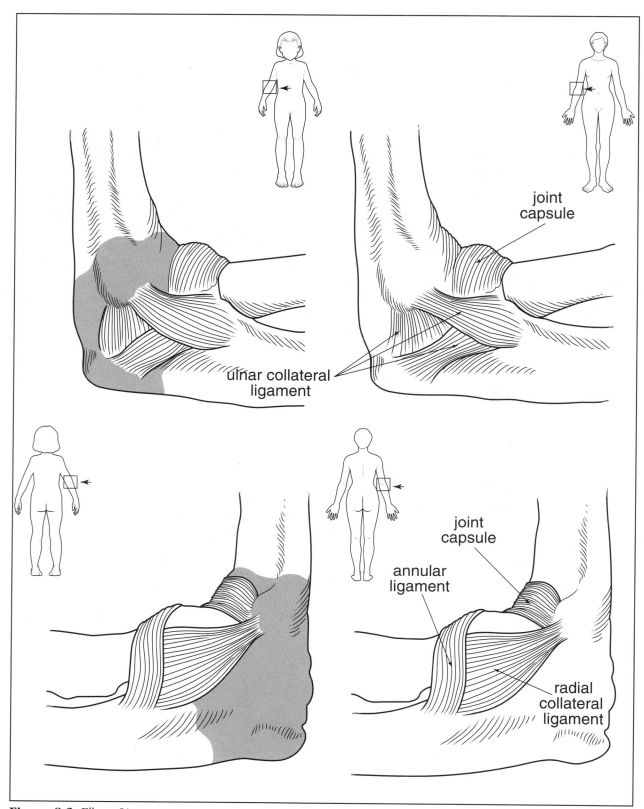

Figure 8.2. Elbow Ligaments

Muscular System

The biceps brachii is frequently implicated as the cause of elbow flexion and pronation contracture in children with cerebral palsy. However, the bicep is a supinator and a contracture occurs throughout the muscle's actions, so it cannot be the cause of the pronation component in the child with cerebral palsy. Lack of joint flexibility must also be ruled out as a contributing factor in the limited range of motion.

Table 8.2
Elbow Muscle Flexibility Testing for Children with Cerebral Palsy

Muscle Group	Testing Technique
Flexors	Stabilize the scapula and extend both the shoulder and the elbow.
Extensors	Stabilize the scapula and flex both the shoulder and the elbow.
Supinators	Stabilize the humerus and pronate the forearm.
Pronators	Stabilize the humerus and supinate the forearm.

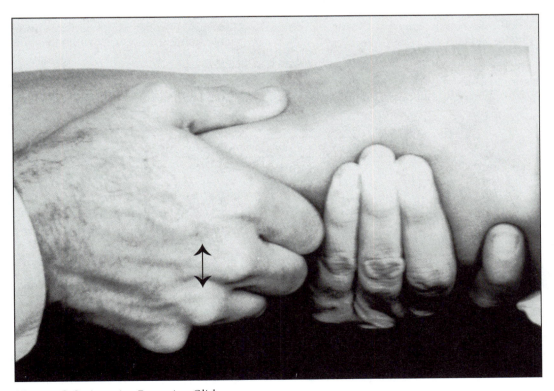

Figure 8.3. Anterior-Posterior Glide
Reproduced by permission of The Saunders Group, Inc. © 1996

Obtaining the range of motion for extension and supination is simple once the joint connective tissue is stretched. However, gaining strength in the new range is a far more difficult task, because very few functional activities involve full supination. Functional tasks tend to occur in pronation, or midway between supination and pronation. The child unable to actively supinate once the range has been obtained may need to begin strengthening with isometric contractions and work up to eccentric and concentric contractions. Isometric contractions while holding objects such as a lightweight paper cup and ice in the involved hand while the child pours water or juice into the cup, tend to be both functional and hold the child's interest. The amount the child can hold (the cup, the cup plus ice, the cup plus ice plus a little water) is an indication of the isometric strength of the muscle. Drinking the contents can be an immediate reward and will also decrease the resistance when necessary.

Table 8.3
Proposed Strength Criteria for Elbow Muscles

Strength Criteria	Flexors	Extensors	Pronators
Poor (movement with gravity eliminated)	Hand to mouth in prone.	Extends elbow along support in prone.	Supinate, pronate in dependent position.
Fair (Movement against gravity)	Hand to mouth in supine.	Reaches in prone.	Supinate, pronate with elbow flexed.
Good (Movement against gravity and some resistance)	Toy to mouth.	Reaches in prone while holding a toy.	Supinate and pronate with elbow flexed and toy in hand.
Normal (Age-appropriate resistance)	Lifts age-appropriate toys.	Reaches in prone while holding age-appropriate toy.	Reaches in prone while holding age-appropriate toy against age-appropriate resistance.
At 3 months	Attempts to bring hand to mouth	Thrusts arm in play	N.A.
At 6 months	Mouths toys	Elevates self by arms in prone	Turns hand in front of face
At 9 months	N.A.	N.A.	N.A.
At 12 months	Holds a ball	N.A.	Bangs spoon with supination
At 18 months	N.A.	Throws a ball	N.A.
At 24 months	N.A.	N.A.	N.A.
At 36 months	N.A.	N.A.	Pours

N.A. Not available. Unable to infer from standardized assessments.

Treatment Planning

Pronated and Flexed Elbow "Flexion Contracture"

Many children with cerebral palsy have an elbow flexion, pronation contracture. Although the biceps are frequently implicated as a causal factor, again, they are supinators and therefore cannot cause the pronation component. Frequently, the cause is limited mobility of the radial head on the humerus and ulna. Increasing flexibility of the periarticular connective tissue around this joint frequently produces increased range.

Table 8.4
Common Evaluation Results and Treatment Options for Elbow Flexion Contracture

System	Findings	Treatment Options
Skeletal	Fusion	None
Ligamentous	Limited mobility in the connective tissue around the superior radial ulnar joint	Mobilize the superior radial ulnar joint.
	Distal radial ulnar joint is seldom a problem.	Leave alone.
Muscular	Weakness in the supinators, especially	Strengthen the supinators and extensors.

Summary

Children with cerebral palsy commonly have limitation to elbow supination and extension. Classically, the biceps brachii are blamed for this situation. However, because the biceps are supinators, contracture of the biceps cannot account for the pronation contracture. Limitation to the motion at the superior radial ulnar joint can produce the characteristic limitation and should be assessed and treated if necessary.

Chapter 9
Wrist and Hand

The wrist controls the length and tension relationships in the multiarticular hand muscles. Because these muscles do not insert on each of the carpal bones, ligamentous integrity is paramount to correct bone alignment during movement.

Skeletal System

The bones of the wrist are the capitate, scaphoid, lunate, triquetrum, pisiform, hamate, trapezoid, and trapezium.

It has been reported that 18- to 36-month-old children have 80 degrees of palmarflexion, 70 degrees of dorsiflexion, 20 degrees of radial deviation, and 30 degrees of ulnar deviation. Babies may crawl with their shoulders internally rotated, requiring only 70 degrees of dorsiflexion, instead of in true quadruped requiring 90 degrees of wrist dorsiflexion, because they do not have 90 degrees of wrist dorsiflexion.

Ligamentous System

The ligaments of the wrist control carpal motion sequence. This in turn produces wrist motion (Mayfield et al. 1976). Excessive mobility in the ligaments produces abnormal range and often subluxations. Too little mobility can directly impair range of motion. The primary ligaments of the wrist are the ulnar and radial collateral, dorsal, and volar radiocarpal and ulnocarpal ligaments (see Figure 9.1).

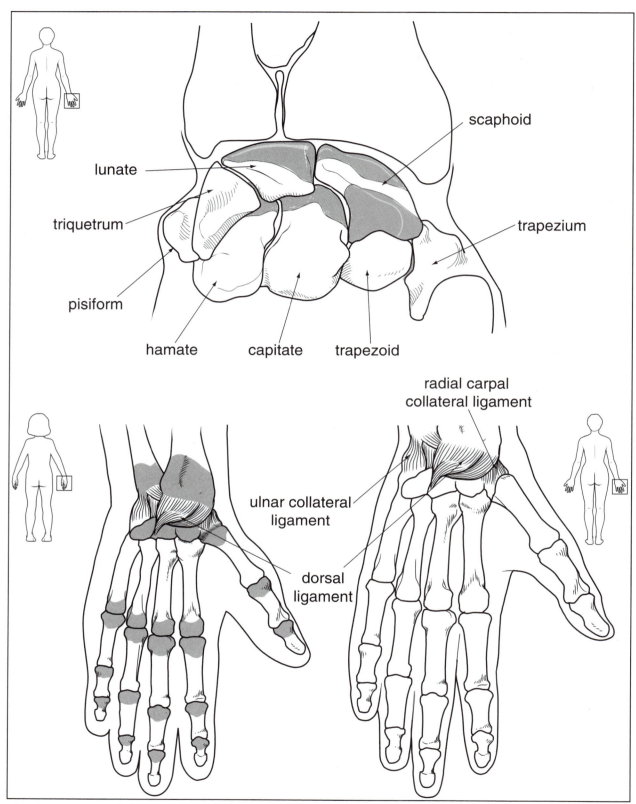

Figure 9.1. Wrist Skeletal System

Radial deviation occurs between the radius and the proximal row of carpals and is a convex on concave action. If the wrist is stuck in ulnar deviation, as in many children with cerebral palsy, the proximal row of carpals is oscillated ulnarly to increase radial deviation.

Palmar- and dorsiflexion occur in sequence. Although the muscles create tension and therefore pull the bones, the ligaments guide the resultant action. The capitate moves palmarly on the scaphoid from full palmarflexion to neutral where the joint becomes close-packed. The scaphoid then moves dorsally on the lunate from neutral to mid dorsiflexion at which point this articulation is close-packed (Figure 9.3). From there to full range of motion, the scaphoid moves palmarly on the radius.

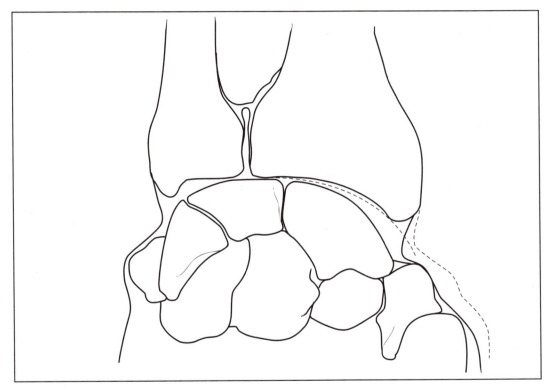

Figure 9.2. Radial Deviation

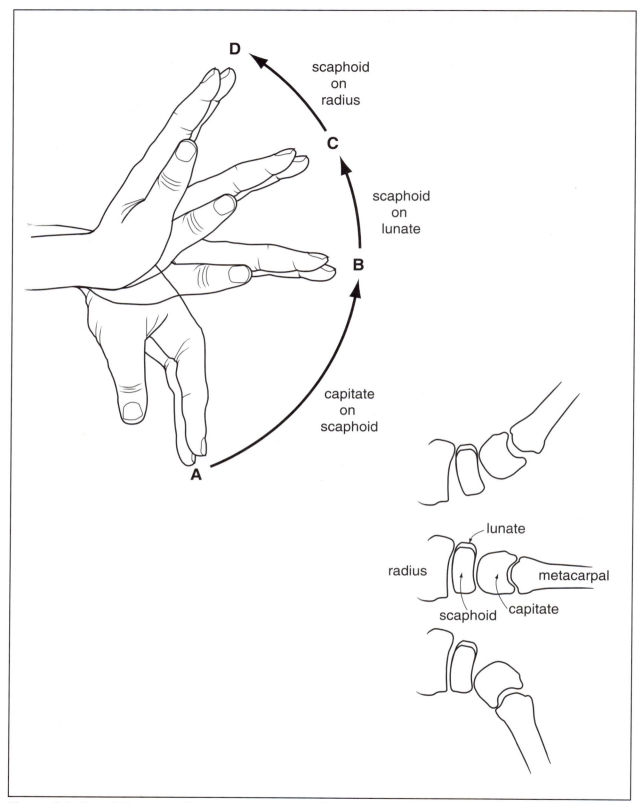

Figure 9.3. Carpal Movement Sequence in Wrist Dorsiflexion

Passive range of motion does not guarantee that this sequence occurs. Consequently, individual joint mobility is a prerequisite to global passive range of motion and muscle flexibility assessment.

Table 9.1 lists and describes techniques to assess ligamentous flexibility in the wrist, and Figures 9.4 to 9.7 illustrate hand placement.

Table 9.1
Techniques to Assess Wrist Ligament Flexibility

Range	Technique	Hand Position	Force Direction
Radial deviation	Ulnar glide	Stabilize the radius and ulna, mobilize the proximal row of carpals	Ulnarly
Ulnar deviation	Radial glide	Stabilize the radius and ulna, mobilize the proximal row of carpals	Radially
Wrist extension	Individual joint mobility	From full palmar flexion to neutral; stabilize the scaphoid and move the capitate	Palmarly
		From neutral to mid-dorsiflexion; stabilize the lunate and move the scaphoid	Dorsally
		From mid to full dorsiflexion, stabilize the radius and move the scaphoid	Palmarly

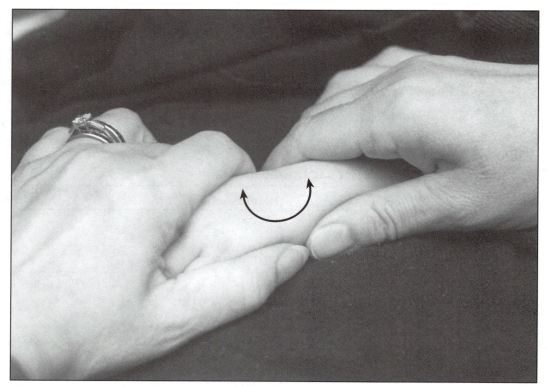

Figure 9.4. Lateral Tilt

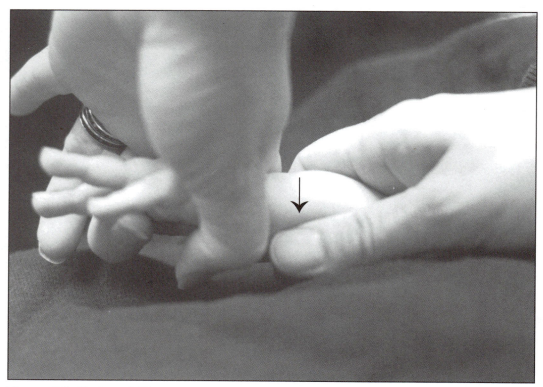

Figure 9.5. Backward Tilt

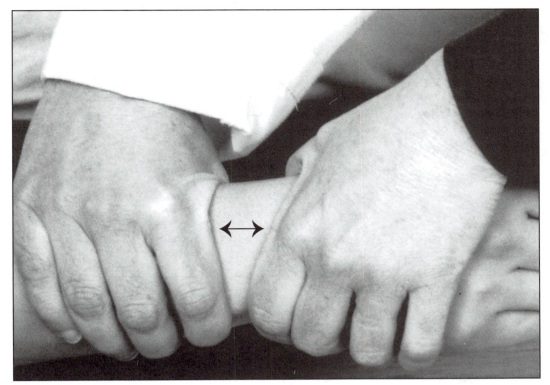

Figure 9.6. Traction
Reproduced by permission of The Saunders Group, Inc. © 1996

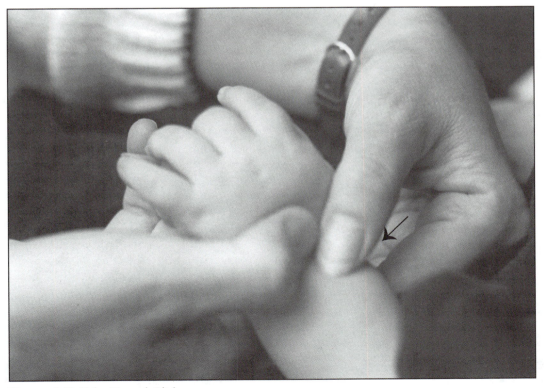

Figure 9.7. Volar/Dorsal Glide

Muscular System

Although individual muscle strength is critical for function, balance between the flexors and extensors is crucial for coordination and control. Imbalance in strength prevents the wrist from completing its function (i.e., to control the length tension relationships in the multiarticular hand muscles).

Because the radial and ulnar deviators are each composed of one flexor and one extensor, tests for flexor and extensor strength also indicate deviator strength.

Table 9.2
Proposed Strength Criteria for Wrist Muscles

Strength Criteria	Flexors	Extensors
Poor (Movement with gravity eliminated)	—	—
Fair (Movement against gravity)	Flexes wrist against gravity, bringing fingers to the mouth.	—
Good (Movement against gravity and some resistance)	Flexes wrist to bring toy to mouth.	—
Normal (Age-appropriate resistance)	Flexes wrist against age-appropriate resistance.	N.A.
At 3 months	N.A.	Keeps hands open.
At 6 months	Grasps rod.	Rotates wrist.
At 9 months	N.A.	Uses finger pads to grasp cube.
At 12 months	N.A.	N.A.
At 18 months	N.A.	N.A.
At 24 months	N.A.	N.A.
At 36 months	Imitates hand movements.	Imitates hand movements.

N.A. Not available. Unable to infer from standardized assessments.

Stabilization of the wrist is critical for hand function. Using the fingers for writing, dressing, or even self-feeding requires the wrist musculature to maintain alignment of the carpals for repetitive motion over prolonged periods of time. One problem in treatment carryover may be that the child can contract the muscle appropriately for two or three repetitions but cannot, for example, continue the contractions through a whole feeding.

Flexibility testing of the wrist musculature assumes normal mobility in the carpals. In children with cerebral palsy, this assumption must be tested to assure muscle flexibility is not obtained at the expense of ligamentous integrity. After assessing the ligaments, maintain wrist extension while stretching the finger flexors over the appropriately aligned carpals. Take care to determine that full muscle flexibility is desired, because maintenance of some flexion may allow the child tenodesis for function.

Treatment Planning

Common wrist problems for children with cerebral palsy have already been described. Table 9.3 charts the evaluation and treatment options to address ulnar deviation and fixed wrist flexion.

Table 9.3
Common Evaluation Results and Treatment Options in the Palmar-Flexed Wrist

System	Findings	Options
Skeletal	Subluxed carpal(s)	Brace.
Ligamentous	Hypermobile joints	Brace or surgery.
	Hypomobile joints in one or more parts of the movement sequence	Mobilize the appropriate joints at the appropriate points in range.
Muscular	Weakness of the flexors and extensors, especially on the radial side	Strengthen as appropriate.
	Limited flexibility	Stretch unless tenodesis is desired.

Summary

The ligamentous system of the wrist is critical to control the motion of the carpals for normal movement. The characteristic movement pattern of the carpals in flexion and extension of the wrist must be assessed and treated if necessary before assessment of finger flexor flexibility.

Children with cerebral palsy frequently have limited motion at the carpals, preventing the normal sequence of movements during flexion and extension of the wrist.

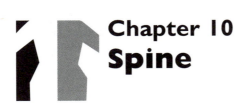

Chapter 10
Spine

Skeletal System

The spine at birth is *c*-curved with the convexity posterior (Figure 10.1). The primary curves therefore are the thoracic and sacral curves, which are convex. The secondary curves are concave posterior; they are the cervical and lumbar curves. The cervical curve develops before birth—as seen on ultrasound—and indeed, it is needed to allow the necessary range for childbirth. The lumbar curve develops as the infant attempts to raise the head up against gravity, which can only be done by reversing the lumbar curve. Lack of range in this area is frequently seen in children with cerebral palsy.

As with many other joints, there is very little documented normal range of motion in the spine for children. The change in range seen in one child over time can be observed in the illustrations of the child in the next chapter.

The spine is composed of a variety of joints including occipital vertebral, C1 on C2, costovertebral and common facet joints. Occipital vertebral and C1 on C2 joints are not generally limited in the child with cerebral palsy. Because management of those joints is so specialized, they will not be addressed in this text. Costovertebral joints are the articulations between the rib and its adjacent vertebrae. Movement here is critical for breathing. These joints often become limited after thoracic surgery, a procedure common with prematurely born infants.

Facet joints vary, and are supported by the intrasegmental (which join adjacent vertebra) and intersegmental (which join several vertebrae) systems (Figure 10.2). The cervical facets are angled between horizontal and coronal planes, gradually changing to coronal in the thoracic spine and shifting to sagittal in the lumbar spine. The average facet joint gradually changes the orientation of its joints. Two joints in the spine, known as the transition vertebrae, show a more marked change between their upper and lower facets than the others. They tend to be C5 or C6 in the neck and between T10 and L2, usually T12 or L1 in the back.

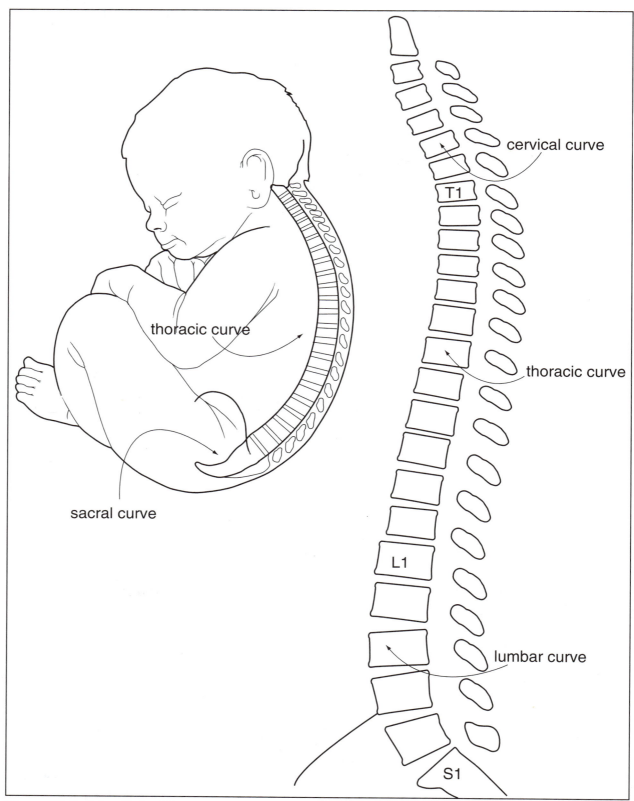

Figure 10.1. Spine Skeletal System

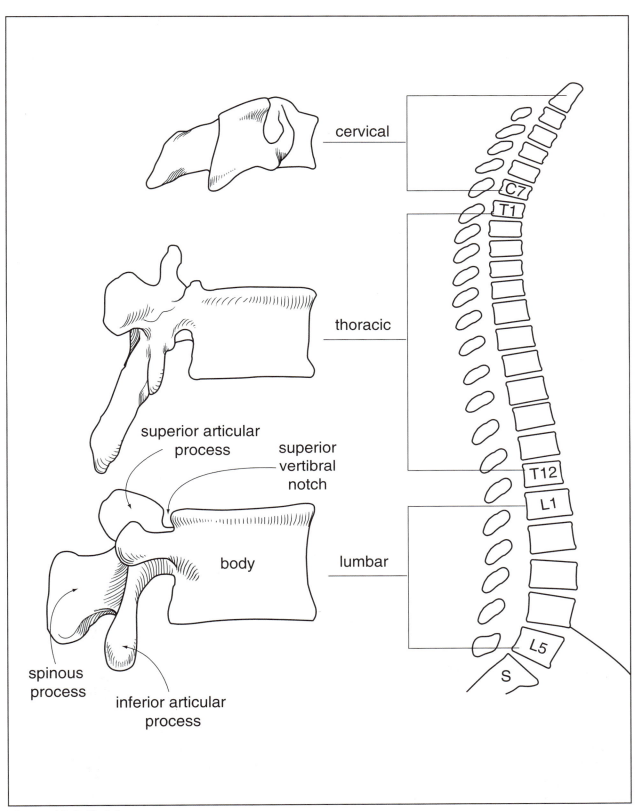

cervical

thoracic

superior articular
process

superior
vertibral
notch

body

lumbar

spinous
process

inferior articular
process

C7
T1
T12
L1
L5
S

Figure 10.2. Vertebrae

These joints allow considerable range because of their multiple orientations. It is interesting that although the spine in the child with cerebral palsy tends to be hypomobile, the transition joints tend to be hypermobile.

Joint Mobility

Motion available in the joints includes flexion, extension, rotation, and lateral flexion. Flexibility for rotation appears when extension is present, usually at about 3 to 4 months of age. Flexibility and strength changes occur together. Rotation and lateral flexion always occur together. This arrangement has a mechanical role in balance. Specifically, when the spine is extended, the upper spine rotates with lateral flexion to the same side, and the lower spine rotates with lateral flexion to the opposite side. In spinal flexion, rotation with lateral flexion can occur to the same side throughout the spine. In spinal extension, rotation of the spine (as in reaching to the right) produces lateral flexion to the right in the neck but lateral flexion to the left in the lumbar spine. The net effect is a maintenance of the center of gravity over the base of support. In spinal flexion, however, rotation to the right allows lateral flexion to the right throughout the spine. This is apparent when watching children with cerebral palsy reach to one side. They can reach down and to one side, but cannot reach up and to the side.

Ligamentous System

The spine is supported by an extensive ligamentous system. The child with cerebral palsy frequently has a kyphosed or, at best, a flat lumbar spine, either of which is flexion of the joints. Spinal extension is frequently limited in the lumbar spine due to ligamentous tightness. If the child is unable to actively extend the lower back, the ligaments can be stretched when the joint is mobilized. In contrast to adult mobilization, gentle broad stretching is indicated. To assess or stretch the connective tissue, place the side of the hand on the child's spinous processes. Take up the slack and oscillate at the end of the joint play to increase extension.

Muscular System

At birth, the back extensors are apparently stretched and the flexors are apparently shortened. Along with achieving flexibility, infants show strength through the range of motion. The infant begins strengthening the neck muscles by raising his head from mom's shoulder to vertical. Gradually, additional antigravity range occurs as the infant then spends the next 3 months attaining enough antigravity strength to assume pivot prone. By 6 to 8 months, the infant can extend the back full range antigravity in sitting.

Table 10.1
Proposed Strength Criteria for Spinal Muscles

Strength Criteria	Flexors	Extensors
Poor (Movement with gravity eliminated)	Trunk flexion in sidelying	Sidelying back extension
Fair (Movement against gravity)	Partial range antigravity, i.e., feet come up	Partial range antigravity, i.e., pivot prone but cannot extend in sitting for a 9-month-old
Good (Movement against gravity and some resistance)	Full range but only partial resistance, i.e., can get feet to mouth but not with shoes on	Full range antigravity but not with age-appropriate resistance, i.e., can get to sitting, but not while holding a toy at 12 months.
Normal (Age-appropriate resistance)	—	—
At 3 months	Feet to mouth.	Head up, steady in vertical; head up in prone.
At 6 months	Turns from back to side.	Sits alone while playing with toy.
At 9 months	Rotates while sitting.	Rotates while sitting.
At 12 months	N.A.	N.A.
At 18 months	N.A.	N.A.
At 24 months	N.A.	N.A.
At 36 months	Lift interior angle of scapula off support (hips at 90°, knees at 120° —per Romero)	
At 48 months	N.A.	N.A.
At 60 months	Lift head and shoulder 90°.	N.A.
At 72 months	N.A.	N.A.

N.A. Not available. Unable to infer from standardized assessments.

Treatment Planning

Kyphotic Lumbar Spine and Head Control

Head control is a common concern in children with cerebral palsy. Often the child is only able to move the head by throwing it posteriorly. Head control in prone is a function of the lumbar spine extension, because normally the cervical spine in head up in prone is flexed. Lumbar joint extension, muscle flexibility, and muscle strength are necessary for head up in prone. Primarily, however, flexibility and strength begin in vertical because the necessary amount of strength against gravity has not developed. This may be why infants achieve head up in prone in vertical (at mom's shoulder) months before they achieve it in prone (Bailey 1993). Once strength and range are achieved in vertical, then they can be achieved in prone.

This principle of close-packed lumbar extension to support the head can be applied to seating and orthotics. Flat-backed wheelchairs encourage kyphosis, especially if the child has less than 90 degrees of hip flexion. The head in kyphosis must be slumped forward or "stacked" back on the neck. A lumbar roll placed in the lumbar part of the back support, coupled with enough hip flexion, places the spine in a more mechanically supportive position. This same principle applies to the molded body jackets designed to prevent scoliosis. The flat-backed jackets do not lock the lumbar spine in close-pack. Molding a lumbar support into the jacket sometimes assists in locking the spine and supporting the head.

Summary

The spine is c-curved at birth with secondary curves developing for specific functions. The cervical secondary curve develops before birth, facilitating normal delivery. The lumbar curve develops as weight is shifted with backward oscillatory movement to result in head up in prone.

Once full extension is present, rotation and lateral flexion can occur. Because of the orientation of the facet joints, rotation and lateral flexion (when they occur in extension) occur in a characteristic pattern that maintains the center of gravity over the base of support with minimal muscular effort. Because children with cerebral palsy seldom have full spinal extension, the normal interaction of rotation and lateral flexion seldom occurs. Consequently, these children require more muscular effort to balance the trunk during movement.

Chapter 11
Skill Development

The acquisition of gross and fine motor skills has been relatively well documented in such work as the Denver Developmental Scales, Gesell Scales, and Peabody Gross and Fine Motor Scales (Bailey 1993; Folio and Fewel 1983; Frankel 1973). However, scales such as the Denver were developed to identify early indicators of mental retardation, not motor control problems (Frankel 1973). This is disconcerting given the amount of therapy prescribed based on motor delays identified by these types of tests alone. The tests can document the delay but they cannot identify the cause of the delay. The therapy evaluation must determine if the delay is due to muscular, skeletal, or neurological factors, and if the delay is amenable to therapy.

Although some variability has been recorded in different scales, the general principle is one of orderly development of neural maturation causing skill acquisition. This principle has been challenged in several ways. First, the timing of skill appearance has changed in this culture since Gesell originally developed the scales, hence the need for revision. Second, it is well established that not all normal children display the same pattern of development. For example, not all non-neurologically involved children crawl before they walk (Bottos et al. 1989; Robson 1984). Third, different ethnic groups display differing rates of motor development (Malina 1988). Fourth, different nationalities display differing sequence and timing of motor milestones (Super 1976; Thornton 1992). An intact neuromusculoskeletal system and practice on a skill seems to be most important to the acquisition of the skill, not how early nor in what sequence the skill appears.

Integration for Skill Acquisition

This section focuses on the integration of neurological, orthopedic, and muscular systems that are prerequisites to motor skills performance.

The classical theories of motor development emphasize that the neurological connections must be present to express the skill. This is aptly illustrated by motor skill delays in the child with mental retardation lacking any other neuromotor problem. All the systems must be functioning correctly, however, for a child to express motor skills with the appropriate quality of movement characteristic of efficient function. For example, a child with spinal muscular atrophy may not practice pivot prone, and a child with arthrogryposis might never get to sit or crawl normally, yet both are neurologically intact.

Skill acquisition and performance have been related to myelination and synaptic maturation. However, skill acquisition and performance have not been related to the musculoskeletal prerequisites required to express the skill. This discussion focuses on the relationship between musculoskeletal prerequisites and skill. Infants gain range and strength on their own. To gain range, infants must stretch the connective tissue elements limiting that range. This is clearly seen in stretching hip connective tissue needed for the hip extension (Lee 1977). Infant movements are characteristically oscillatory and at the end of their available range. As the oscillations stretch the tissue, children continue oscillatory movements, now in a new range. The oscillatory movements at the end of joint range require repetitive contraction and relaxation of the muscles. Infants continue this pattern of oscillating near the end range, adding appropriate resistance to gain strength in the new range.

Children gain new range through oscillatory movements and add resistance to the oscillations to increase strength. Infants can increase resistance in two ways. First, an increase in the lever arm is an increase in resistance. As a child initially gains control for reach in prone, sitting, or standing, the arms are in high guard. That is, they are abducted from the body in the coronal plane, bringing the center of gravity over the base of support. As strength develops, muscular resistance increases by extending the elbow. Second, strength develops during play with weights, such as toys. An infant will pick up the rattle but not a teddy bear, and an older child will pick up a teddy bear but not a push toy. The weight of the toy is a measure of the resistance available to the muscle. Standard children's toys can be weighed and used as objective measures of strength in the clinical setting. Combining increased levers and weights provides strength in function, such as in reaching and throwing.

Pictorial Sequence of Development

The following pictorial sequence of development illustrates these points in a given child. The figures are illustrations of one normally developing child drawn from monthly photographs taken as she matured. A detailed examination of the illustrations suggests strength and range changes over time combined with neurological maturation are all necessary for a skill to appear.

Head Control

Head control in prone is one of the first skills to emerge. Lacey et al. (1985) observed 104 infants, 25 to 33 weeks gestational age. They identified a pattern of head side turning that decreased spinal extension; however, the central position of the head required more spinal extension. At 35 to 39 weeks post-conceptual age, the 11 infants with later motor handicap showed a persistence of decreased spinal extension.

Comparing Figure 11.1 (1-week-old, full-term child) and Figure 11.2 (the same child at 1 month), note the flexed spine with head to side consistent with the description of Lacey et al. (1985). Note that by 2 months (Figure 11.3), significant increases in lumbar spine and hip extension are evident. The hip extension changes are consistent with research on changes in hip range of motion previously reported. For the head to come up prone and keep the eyes level, the cervical spine is flexed. To bring the head up, the increased lumbar extension appears necessary. Figures 11.4 and 11.5 illustrate the continuing increase in lumbar extension through 11 months. Figure 11.4 shows a marked increase in the thoracolumbar junction but not a smooth curve throughout the lumbar spine. By 11 months (Figure 11.5), extension occurs throughout the lumbar spine.

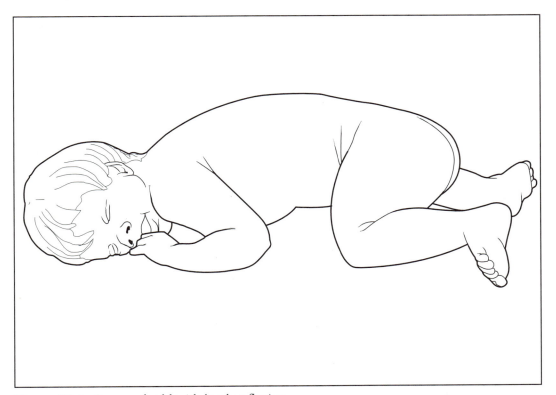

Figure 11.1. One-week-old with lumbar flexion

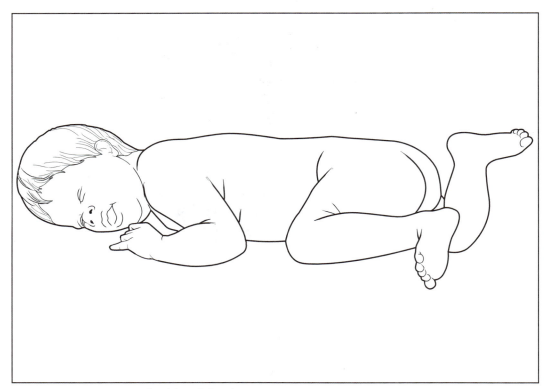

Figure 11.2. One-month-old with lumbar extension

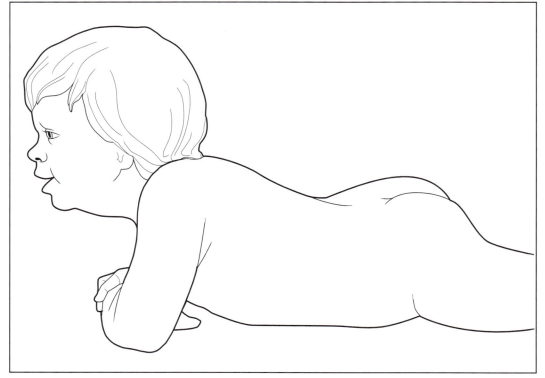

Figure 11.3. Two-month-old with lumbar extension

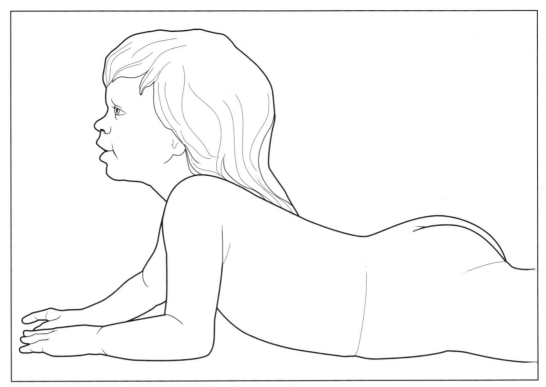

Figure 11.4. Nine-month-old with lumbar extension

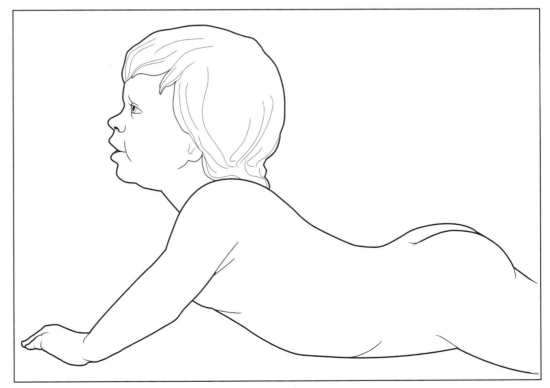

Figure 11.5. Eleven-month-old with lumbar extension

To achieve head up in prone, it appears that the normal infant must shift his or her head and oscillate weight backwards. This weight shift may provide the force necessary to increase the connective tissue flexibility for lumbar spine and hip extension. This in turn increases range and provides the repetition necessary to gain strength and influence neural stability. The child with neurological compromise does not appear to be able to change the range and strength for normal motor performance (Lacey et al. 1985, among others). Muscular weakness preventing the head to come to midline, or oscillate sufficiently while it is there, may lead to failure of the spine and hips to increase their range. This failure to increase range and subsequently strength in the range prevents appropriate joint mobility for movement of the center of gravity over the base of support in future skills. This failure to increase range to normal values often appears later as a contracture. Perhaps the contracture in older children with neurological damage did not develop, but was maintained from infancy. The hip contracture "normal" in the infant is "abnormal" in the older child with cerebral palsy.

Reach

Oscillation of the head and weight shift toward the posterior is a pattern repeated throughout normal development. Progressing from head up in prone described above, as the oscillations continue in neurologically intact children, swimming or pivot prone occurs. This brings the arms from the surface but keeps them near the body. Yet reaching out requires more range and strength through the shoulder girdle due to the increased length of the lever arm. Thelen et al. (1993) studied reaching in the infant and concluded that reaching appears between 12 and 22 weeks. Thelen notes that reaching appears when an infant can intentionally adjust force and compliance of the arm, often using muscle coactivation. These patterns are therefore consequences of the match between system dynamics and the task (Thelen et al. 1993). The natural dynamic of the system includes the available range and strength.

At birth, the arms cannot reach this high guard position in pivot prone, nor reach for objects. Range and strength must be increased for high guard in pivot prone or reaching. In the pictorial example explored here, initially the little girl had about 60 degrees of shoulder elevation (Figure 11.6). As the little girl increased her head up relative to prone, she continued to oscillate and shift her weight backward with the arms on the support. The child continues this oscillatory posterior weight shift across the sternoclavicular joints. Consistent with the function of the sternoclavicular joints, increasing joint range will allow the infant to raise the arm from its initial 60 degree (approximately) abduction and flexion to approximately 100 degrees necessary for prone on hands and reaching. She showed active shoulder range of less than 90 degrees at 1 month of age (Figure 11.7), progressing to slightly more than 90 degrees at 2 months (Figure 11.8). By 6 months, she can reach forward approximately 110 degrees (Figure 11.9). Note the normal side position of the scapula as she reaches. It is unclear when the full adult range of shoulder elevation is achieved. If the acromioclavicular joint is a fibrocartilagenous union until approximately 2 years of age, as some suggest (Cailliet 1966), it cannot contribute to "normal" scapulohumeral rhythm. Consequently, it is possible the adult norm of 170 degrees of flexion and abduction is not achieved until after 2 years. This observation was verified by Freedman and Munroe (1966) and Doody and Waterland (1970). If it is accurate, then implications for passive range of motion exercises, placing baby prone over bolsters and wedges, and potential overstretching of the glenohumeral joint in children with cerebral palsy are obvious considerations.

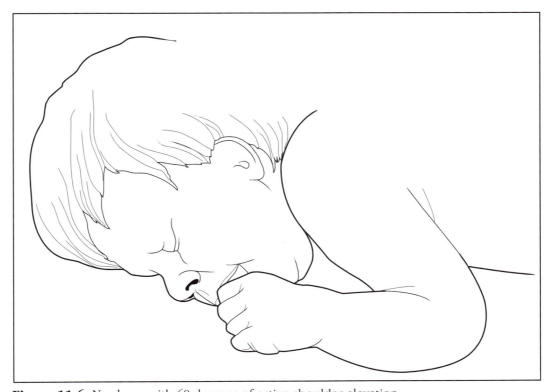

Figure 11.6. Newborn with 60 degrees of active shoulder elevation

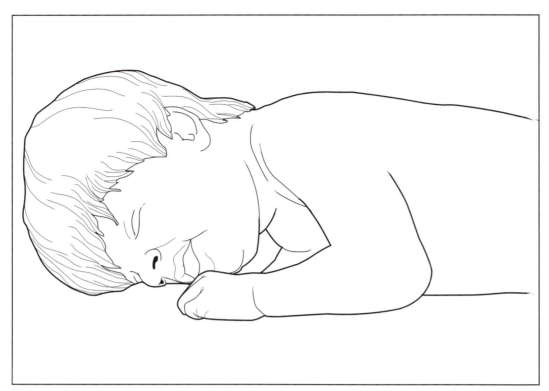

Figure 11.7. One-month-old with less than 90 degrees of active shoulder range

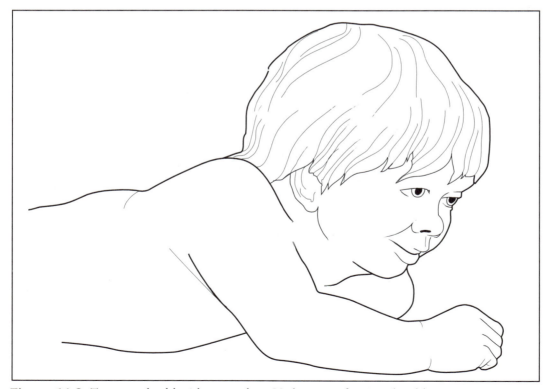

Figure 11.8. Two-month-old with more than 90 degrees of active shoulder range

This pattern of weight shifting posteriorly and oscillating across various joints to gain range and ultimately strength reappears as infants achieve sitting. Contrary to the frequently taught pattern of rolling from supine to the side to push up into sitting, getting into sitting appears to be a continuation of the pattern to shift the center of gravity backwards. The child in this pictorial example illustrates a common method children use to get to sit. She starts in prone and pulls her knee up under or along the side of her trunk, then pushes backward over the flexed leg (Figures 11.10 to 11.12). Most children with cerebral palsy cannot flex the hip adequately for this task, nor push their body weight backwards over the other leg. They frequently do not have the range and strength necessary to perform the task in this way.

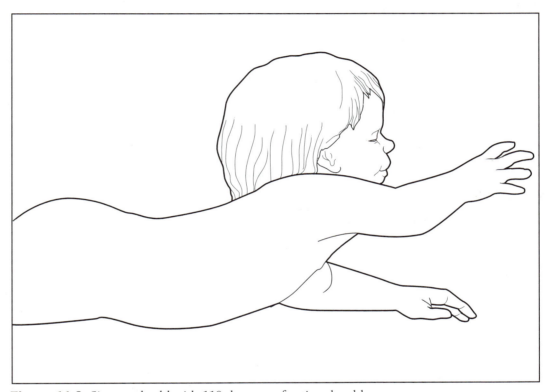

Figure 11.9. Six-month-old with 110 degrees of active shoulder range

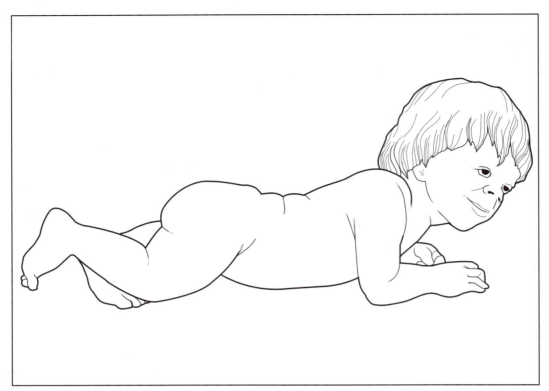

Figure 11.10. Get to sit I

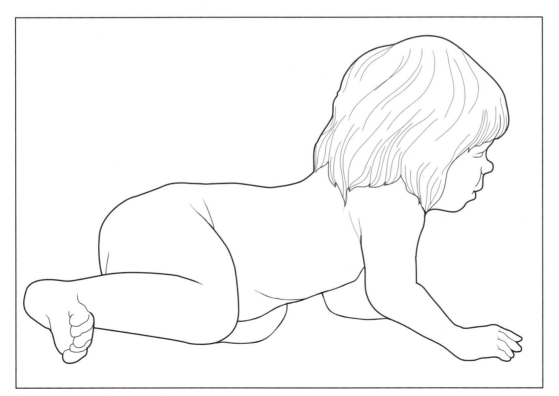

Figure 11.11. Get to sit II

Sitting Sequence

The sitting sequence illustrates how range can be present for back extension (as in pivot prone), though not shown due to an inability of the child to raise the trunk full range antigravity. At 1 month (Figure 11.13), the child in the illustration shows the completely rounded back in a pull to sit maneuver. By 2 months (Figure 11.14), the infant sits slumped forward with only minimal extension in the lumbar spine. Again, the pattern of oscillating the center of gravity backwards is repeated as the child tries to come up into straight sitting. By 6 months (Figure 11.15), the child has enough extension to sit with a straight back. Note that this range existed previously in prone but is only now seen in upright. Possibly strength has improved so that back extensors can bring the longer lever of the extended back up through the full range of motion against gravity. Once the spine achieves closed pack, only minimal strength is necessary to maintain the posture. Between 6 and 7 months this child continues to gain strength in the hamstrings and back extensors by increasing the distance of the arm from the trunk and adds the weight of a toy, as seen as the child shifts her head back over the pelvis, brings arms forward toward the knees (Figure 11.16), and holds a toy (Figure 11.17).

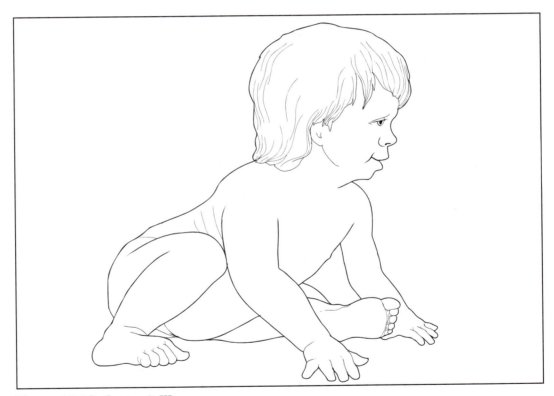

Figure 11.12. Get to sit III

Back extensors control movement from the lumbar spine to the head but do not control the more vertical position of the pelvis over the femurs. Hamstring strength from 90-degree hip flexion forward is necessary to control the center of gravity over the base of support within the pelvis. Continued strength in the back and hamstring muscles is necessary as the child's arms come out of high guard and she begins to hold and throw toys (increasing the levers and resistance).

In contrast to this little girl, children with cerebral palsy show marked differences in range and antigravity strength. For example, very few children with cerebral palsy have greater than 90 degree hip flexion. They cannot get the center of gravity forward over the base of support as our example did in Figure 11.16. With the center of gravity behind the base of support, as in sacral sitting, strength of the back extensors and hamstrings is not needed. Isometric strength of the abdominals and hip flexors is necessary to prevent the child from falling backwards. This may set up the pattern of continued weakness in the back extensors and hamstrings at 90 degrees of hip flexion with concomitant isometric strength of the abdominals and the hip flexors so commonly seen in children with cerebral palsy who sacral-sit. In contrast, children who reverse tailor-sit do use their back extensors and hamstrings to sit. Children who reverse tailor-sit tend to be more mobile in sitting, possibly because they use the muscles eccentrically and concentrically, as opposed to children who sacral-sit.

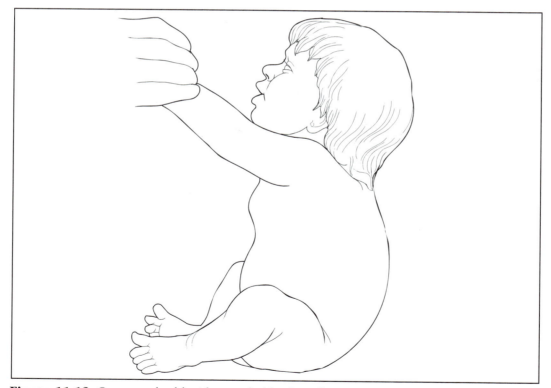

Figure 11.13. One-month-old with rounded back, pull-to-sit maneuver

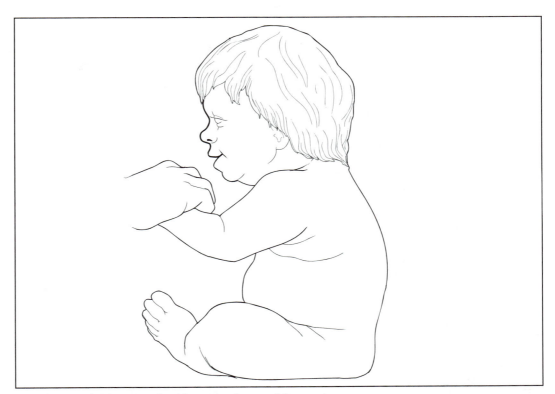

Figure 11.14. Two-month-old sitting slumped forward

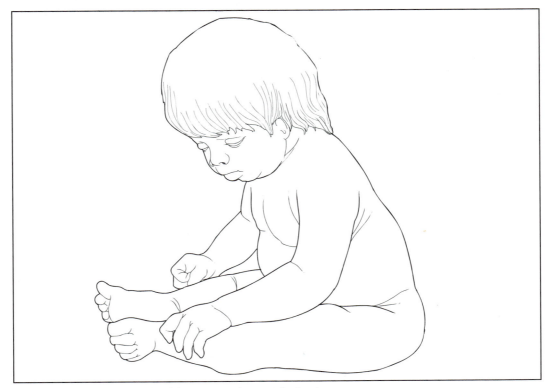

Figure 11.15. Six-month-old sitting with straight back

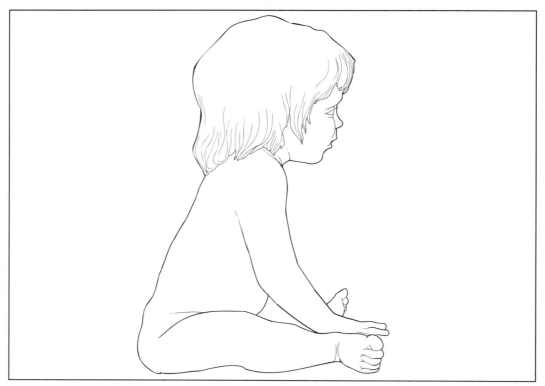

Figure 11.16. Six-month-old shifting head back over pelvis and bringing arms forward toward the knees

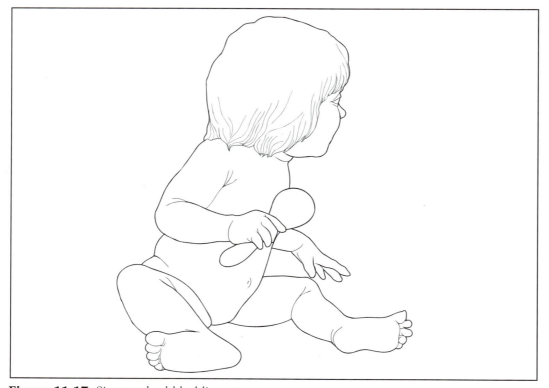

Figure 11.17. Six-month-old holding a toy

Once sitting, neurologically intact children usually try to locomote. Crawling is the next skill in the classic developmental sequence, though it is a controversial movement. Some authors hypothesize crawling is critical for later sensorimotor development (Fabry et al. 1973; McEwan et al. 1991). These studies appear to begin with children with problems and note that many of them had difficulty with motor skills, such as crawling. Other authors used a prospective approach to document development of locomotor skills. Robson (1984) and Bottos et al. (1989) both identified a pattern different from the classic. Robson reported that 82 percent of normal infants crawl in quadruped before walking, leaving 18 percent of the normal population who do not crawl first. Hitching or shuffling in sitting is the next most common form of prewalking locomotion, occurring in 9 percent of the normal population. Only 2 percent of the normal population walk directly from creeping or rolling. Both investigators found similar patterns in that the earliest ambulators not only did not crawl first, but they showed no prewalking locomotor pattern. They simply got up and walked. Bottos et al. (1989) found that prewalking locomotion pattern was not predictive of linguistic or psychomotor development at 5 years of age.

Crawling and Standing

If crawling were required for walking, then crawling would contribute prerequisites for walking. Researchers suggest this is not the case. Dunbar et al. (1986) suggest significant differences in muscle use between quadruped and bipedal locomotion. They observed that quadripedal positioning requires upper extremity coactivation with reciprocal activation of the lower extremity in a proximal to distal pattern. Bipedal positioning, however, shows a distal to proximal muscle pattern to control the center of gravity over the base of support. This distal to proximal muscle pattern is consistent with that observed by Nashner (1976, 1977, 1981) under conditions where feet are fully supported on a stable base. These authors suggest that crawling is not critical for normal neuromotor development of ambulation, and that quadruped locomotion is a very different movement pattern from bipedal locomotion. Given the difficulty most children with cerebral palsy have with crawling, serious consideration should be given in the therapeutic setting to the age of the child and to the time and resources expended on crawling at the expense of walking.

The case has been made that standing is a totally different skill from quadruped, requiring totally different range and strength parameters. Changes in hip, knee, and ankle range are noticeable in the illustration series of the child in this example in moving from supported to independent standing. At 1 month (Figure 11.18), adduction of the lower extremities is common and normal. The hip and knee are flexed with plantarflexed ankles consistent with the limitations of passive range reported in earlier research. However, by 2 months (Figure 11.19), the hip is more extended (though still in some flexion as noted earlier), the knee is extending (but still in some flexion), and the ankle dorsiflexes to begin accepting some weight. By 6 months (Figure 11.20), more weight can be supported by the child, but the hip and knee flexion are still normally present. Again, this is consistent with range changes noted in the research. A bigger range change appears about 8 months (Figure 11.21) in this child. Hips and knees are significantly less flexed, shifting body weight over the base of support. Weight is still slightly forward of the base of support due to the hip flexion.

Walking becomes possible if the base is increased to allow the center of gravity to fall within it. This is seen as children walk with hands held or while using a push toy (Figure 11.22). Finally, as the hip comes into more extension, bringing the center of gravity back over the base of support formed by the pelvis and lower extremities, the child is free to stand (Figure 11.23). Notice in early walkers the progression from high guard to arms at side to holding small toys. This progression certainly suggests an improvement in strength as the resistance of levers and outside weights increase. This is the same pattern seen earlier in sitting.

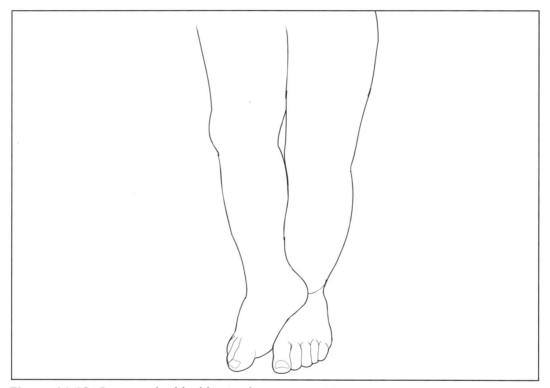

Figure 11.18. One-month-old adducting lower extremities

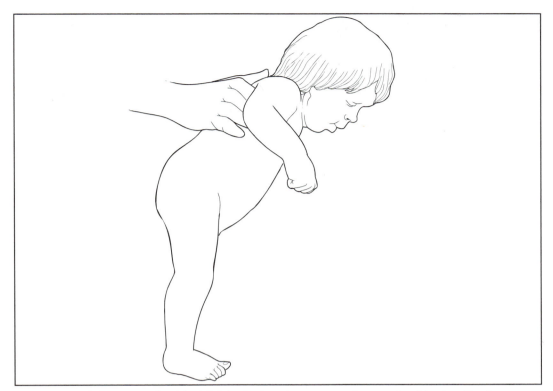

Figure 11.19. Two-month-old with hip flexion, knee extension, and ankle dorsiflexion

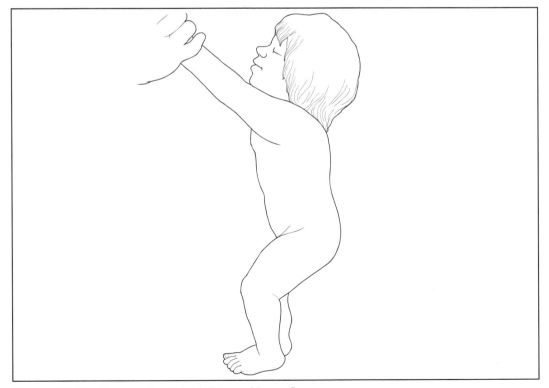

Figure 11.20. Six-month-old with hip and knee flexion

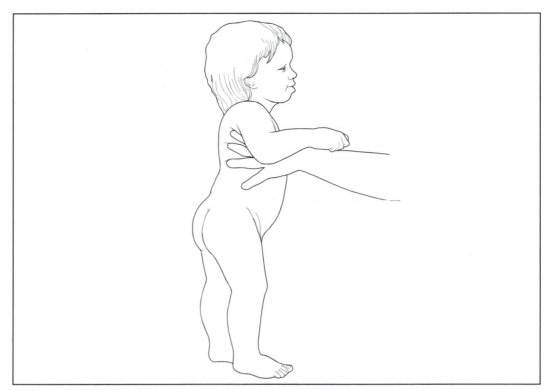

Figure 11.21. Eight-month-old with increased hip and knee flexion

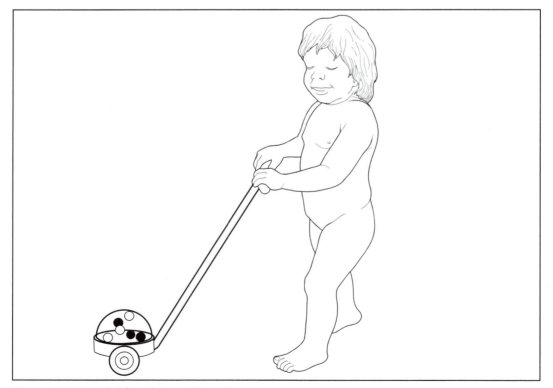

Figure 11.22. Child walking with push toy

Stability in Stance

Standing for children with cerebral palsy frequently maintains the earlier range limitations. The retained range limitations also maintain the center of gravity outside of the base of support and prevent stability in the close-packed position. Either the child with cerebral palsy requires something to hold to ambulate, or compensates in other ways to put the center of gravity over the base of support. This may be accomplished by flexing the knees more to lower the center of gravity, or hyperextending the back to place the center of gravity over the pelvis, even though the hips do not extend enough. Either way, muscular effort for standing is increased and efficiency in standing is compromised. Instead of being able to stand in close-packed position with minimal eccentric and concentric muscle action to adjust sway, the child with cerebral palsy requires isometric muscle action just to maintain standing against gravity. The flexed knee stance requires hamstrings and adductors to isometrically hold the hip up against gravity, quadriceps to isometrically hold the knee, and the gastrocsoleous group to isometrically hold the ankle. It is little wonder that these muscles tend to develop isometric strength in part of their range (Kramer and MacPhail 1994; Rosenflack and Andreasson 1980; Tang and Aymer 1981) but little of the eccentric and concentric strength necessary for efficient movement.

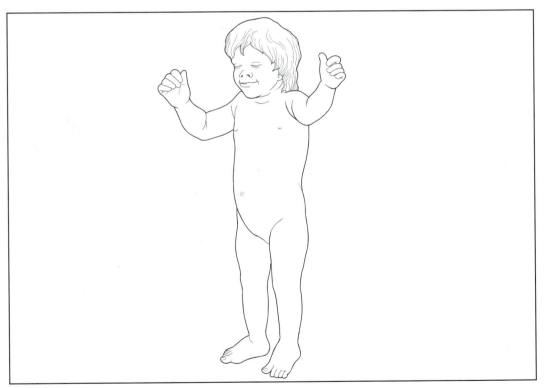

Figure 11.23. Child standing

Balance

Balance has traditionally been considered preplanned or reflexive with set proximal to distal patterns. Researchers have investigated both of these assumptions. Balance appears to be a long loop response to perturbation of the center of gravity over the base of support, which is neither reflexive nor cognitive but based on the situational factors of the time. Several strategies to maintain balance are identified. The ankle strategy utilizes distal to proximal sequencing for low frequency excursions. The hip strategy, on the other hand, occurs in response to high frequency shifts utilizing distal to proximal sequencing. Bending knees and stepping sideways are two other viable strategies to maintain the center of gravity over the base of support (Nashner et al. 1983). Children with spastic hemiplegia, for example, demonstrate normal distal to proximal sequencing in the less involved leg but a variety of disorders in the more involved leg: proximal to distal sequencing, cocontraction, slower onset latency, and variation in amplitude and strength, among others. Children with spastic diplegia, on the other hand, sometimes demonstrate a pattern similar to that seen in hemiplegia but bilaterally, or some have disorganization of the sensory input combination of visual, vestibular, and somatosensory systems as well as disorders of motor coordination (Nashner et al. 1983). Any decrease in range of motion or strength will necessarily affect the balance strategy.

Walking

From standing, walking should allow a highly efficient means of moving the body from one place to another. Sutherland and Cooper (1984) have extensively studied normal gait changes from childhood through adulthood. Table 11.1 summarizes changes in performance criteria at various ages, and Table 11.2 summarizes the changes in range of motion at various ages.

In general, Sutherland et al. (1980) found that gait characteristics change throughout the first 3 years. They change more gradually until about 7 years of age; by 7, the characteristics closely approximate adult patterns. This is consistent with results indicating that muscle patterns in childhood ambulation are variable until 7 to 10 years, when the muscle firing approximates adult patterns. These same observations of childhood variability leading to mature adult patterns are seen in the progression in balance strategies. Sutherland and Cooper (1984) identified specific performance criteria to assess the gait in children. The criteria are width of the base of support, arm swing, initial contact, range of motion, cadence, velocity, step and stride length, swing phase, and stance phase. All but swing phase and stance phase can readily be approximated in a clinical setting. Chalking the shoes while allowing the child to walk down a white paper is a way to clinically measure width of base of support, initial contact, and step and stride length. The addition of a stopwatch allows estimation of cadence and velocity. Range of motion measurements require a goniometer. Arm swing can be observed as present or absent. Norms are presented in Table 11.1. Although these measures are not reliable by research standards, they are more concrete in assessing efficiency in a child's gait than vague references to improved balance or quality. Combining these measures with heart rate and respiratory rates can give an objective clue to the child's overall fitness for ambulation in functional settings such as home or community.

Table 11.1
Performance Criteria

Age	Width of Base of Support	Arm Swing	Initial Contact	Range of Motion	Cadence	Step Length Velocity	Swing Stride Length	Stance Phase	Phase
1 year	Wide	None	Flat Foot	Hip extension, knee extension, ankle extension.	High (175.7 steps/ min.)	Low (63.7 cm/ second) knee extension)	21.6 cm. (43 cm for strike 49.2% mild foot drop)	Opposite toe-off 17.1% (opposite foot 67%)	Single limb 33.5% (toe-off
2 years	Decreasing	Present	Heel strike appearing	Pelvic tilt, external rotation of hip, knee>flexion after strike and before toe-off.	155.8 steps/ minute	71.8 cm/ second (54.9 cm)	27.5 cm (opposite foot strike 50.4% no foot drop)	Opposite toe-off 16.9% (toe-off 67%)	Single limb 33/5%
3 years	Narrow	—	Well-developed heel strike	Adult pattern					
7 years	—	—	—	—	143.5 steps/ minute	114.3 cm/ second (96.5 cm)	47.9 cm 12.4% (opposite foot strike 50%)	Opposite toe-off 37.6% (toe-off 62.4%)	Single limb
Adult	—	—	—	—	114 steps/ minute	121.6 cm/ second (129.4 cm)	65.5 cm 13.4% (Opposite foot strike 50%)	Opposite toe-off 36.7% (toe-off 63.6%)	Single limb

Table 11.2
Range of Motion (Approximate)

Age	Pelvic Rotation	Pelvic Tilt	Hip Rotation	Pelvic Obliquity	Hip Flexion/Extension	Femoral Rotation	Foot Rotation	Knee Flexion/Extension	Knee Rotation	Plantar/Hip Adduction	Dorsi-Flexion	Tibial Rotation
1 year	12" internal, 12" external	18°–22° anterior	10°–30° external	5° up to 5° down	10°–50° flexion	10°–20° external	10°–15° external	10°–65° flexion	5° external to 5° internal	15° abduction to neutral	20° plantar-flexion to 5° dorsiflexion	5°–25° external
2 years	12" internal, 12" external	12°–17°	12° external to 5° internal	3° up to 3° down	50° flexion and 0° extension	5° internal, 15° external	5°–15° external	10°–70° flexion	10° external, 0° internal	10° abduction, 5° adduction	20° plantar-flexion, 10° dorsiflexion	5° internal, 20° external
3 years	12" internal, 12" external	12°–17°	10° external to 5° internal	3° up to 3° down	30° flexion, 0° extension	5° internal, 15° external	5°–15° external	10°–70° flexion	10° external, 0° internal	10° abduction, 5° adduction	20° plantar-flexion, 10° dorsiflexion	5° internal, 20° external
4 years	—	—	—	—	—	—	—	—	—	—	—	—
5 years	—	—	—	—	—	—	—	—	—	—	—	—
6 years	—	—	—	—	—	—	—	—	—	—	—	—
7 years	10" internal, 10" external	13°–17°	10° external, 10° internal	5° up to 5° down	30° flexion, 0° extension	10° internal, 10° external	5°–10° external	10°–70° flexion	10° external, 0° internal	10° abduction, 5° adduction	20° plantar-flexion, 15° dorsiflexion	5° internal, 20° external
Adult	10" internal, 5" external	17°	5° external, 5° internal	5° up, 5° down	30° flexion, 0° extension	8° internal, 8° external	12° external 3° internal	5°–65° flexion	12° external, 0° internal	10° abduction, 0° adduction	20° plantar-flexion, 20° dorsiflexion	5° internal, 20° external

Sutherland and Cooper (1984) carefully documented range necessary in normal movement (Table 11.2). For example, hip flexion and "extension" ranged from 10 to 50 degrees of flexion in the 1-year-old. Given this age does not have full extension range available, this result is consistent. Note that for the next 2 years, however, the child uses less flexion (reducing from 50 to 30 degrees) and goes to full extension. If, as in the child with cerebral palsy, full extension is not possible, increased muscle activity must occur to support the body against gravity and interferes in the expression of the normal determinants of gait.

The Determinants of Gait

The determinants of gait normally limit the excursion of the center of gravity over the base of support, conserving energy from muscular effort. Six determinants control the center of gravity over the base of support, leading to increased efficiency and decreased muscular effort. Children with cerebral palsy frequently lack the range and strength to adequately express the determinants. A review of the determinants of gait from the perspective of range, strength, and speed will be considered.

1. *Lateral pelvic tilt*. Lateral pelvic tilt adjusts length of the leg from pushoff to heel strike. This requires spinal rotation and lateral flexion in spinal extension as well as hip abduction and adduction. Good strength of the abductors in single limb stance, both eccentrically and concentrically, is necessary to support the pelvis through this excursion. Because the child ambulates at approximately 150 steps per minute, the muscle must be able to contract and relax 75 times in a minute!

2. *Knee flexion phase of gait*. Knee flexion adjusts leg length and lowers the center of gravity in stance. Because gait usually requires 15 degrees (or less) of knee flexion in stance, the rotary action of the tibia on the femur is critical to control the knee. Strength of the quadriceps in terminal knee extension and hamstrings to decelerate the knee in swing are necessary for control of the joint. As previously mentioned, speed of contraction and relaxation is considerably greater than the average therapy session.

3. *Knee-ankle interaction*. Knee-ankle interaction shifts weight as rotary forces are absorbed. This determinant requires not only the previous one, but also mobility of the talocrural joint. If one is wearing flat shoes, 5 degrees of dorsiflexion are used to shift the body forward. If wearing heels, flexibility to dorsiflexion is necessary but dorsiflexion is not achieved. Although it is important to have mobility into dorsiflexion, plantar-flexion is also critical for pushoff. Children with no plantarflexion have difficulty propelling the body forward. Both eccentric and concentric strength of the gastroc-soleous group is necessary to control body weight forward and pushoff, respectively. Many children with cerebral palsy, although they stand on their toes (isometric contraction), cannot go up and down on their toes in single limb stance (eccentric-concentric contractions against body weight). These children do not have adequate strength in the plantarflexors to allow control of the tibia in knee-ankle interaction.

4. *Knee-ankle-foot interaction*. Knee-ankle-foot interaction continues the weight shift forward over the foot. The required range, strength, and speed for the previous two determinants is required here with the addition of the foot. The interaction between the subtalor and the midtarsal joints allows mobility to absorb rotary stresses as well

as stability for the rigid lever for push off. Abnormal mobility (either too much or too little) interferes in this normal mechanism. Because this mobility is necessary for ankle strategies in balance, correct mobility here can have a dramatic effect on efficient gait. Strength of the supinators (gastrocsoleous, anterior tibialis, poster tibialis) must be able to tolerate the resistance of the body's weight. Speed in gait was discussed above; however, speed of contraction and relaxation to match age-normal gait speed in this determinant is also critical for standing balance.

5. *Rotation of the pelvis over the fixed femur.* Forward/backward rotation of the pelvis shifts the center of gravity forward. As in the first determinant, this requires spinal extension, rotation and lateral flexion, as well as hip internal and external rotation. This determinant is heavily dependent upon momentum of the swing leg. Because many children with cerebral palsy do not move fast or freely enough to develop momentum, they frequently use muscular effort to shift the center of gravity forward.

6. *Physiological valgus of the knee.* Physiologic valgus of the knee is present or absent, but not amenable to therapy.

Summary

There is little argument that the gait deviations exhibited by children with cerebral palsy are an inefficient means of locomotion from an objective standard, even if the gait exhibited by a given child is the most efficient for that child at that time. The goal of therapy is not to make the gait look better or more normal, but to make it as efficient as possible for that child. The closer children with cerebral palsy come to the normal values for these determinants, the more efficient their gait will be.

As gait and balance are investigated with more sophisticated techniques, and as assumptions can be investigated, the complexity and variability of human movement becomes more apparent. Only through an interaction and cooperation among body systems can efficient movement allow children to express themselves. This manual has presented considerations beyond just the nervous system that affect movement. It is hoped that it will contribute alternative strategies to improve efficient movement in the therapeutic setting.

Bibliography

Akeson, W. H. 1961. An experimental study of joint stiffness. *Journal of Bone and Joint Surgery* 43A:1022–34.

Akeson, W. H., D. Amiel, and D. LaViolette. 1967. The connective tissue response to immobility. *Clinical Orthopedics* 51:1833–97.

Ashton, B., B. Pickles, and J. Roll. 1978. Reliability of goniometric measurements of hip motion in spastic cerebral palsy. *Developmental Medicine and Child Neurology* 20(1): 87–94.

Astbury, J., A. Orgill, B. Bajuk, and V. Ui. 1986. Sequelae of growth failure in appropriate for gestational age, very low birthweight infants. *Developmental Medicine and Child Neurology* 28(4): 472–9.

Astrand, P., and K. Rodahl. 1977. *Textbook of work physiology*. St. Louis, MO: McGraw-Hill.

Badgley, C. 1949. Etiology of congenital dislocation of the hip. *Journal of Bone and Joint Surgery* 31-A: 341–56.

Bar-Or, O. 1983. *Pediatric work physiology*. Berlin: Springer Verlag.

Bartlett, M., L. Wold, D. Shurtleff, L. Staheli. 1985. Hip flexion contractures: A comparison of measurement methods. *Archives of Physical Medicine and Rehabilitation* 66(9): 620–25.

Bailey, N. 1993. *Bailey scales of infant development*. 2d ed. San Antonio, TX: The Psychological Corporation.

Basmajian, J. 1975. *Muscles alive*. Baltimore, MD: Williams & Wilkins.

Beals, R. 1969. Developmental changes in the femur and acetabulum in spastic paraplegia and diplegia. *Developmental Medicine and Child Neurology* 11:303–13.

Bentley, G. 1975. Articular cartilage studies and osteoarthrosis. *Annuals Royal College Surgery England* 57(2):86–199.

Bernhardt, D. 1988. Prenatal and postnatal growth and development of the foot and ankle. *Physical Therapy* 68(12):1831–39.

Bleck, E. 1982. Developmental orthopedics, III: Toddlers. *Developmental Medicine and Child Neurology* 24(4):533–55.

Bleck, E. 1987. *Orthopaedic management in cerebral palsy*. Philadelphia: Lippincott.

Bobath, K. 1980. *A neurophysiological basis for the treatment of cerebral palsy*. Philadelphia: Lippincott.

Bottos, M., B. Dalla, D. Stefani, G. Pettena, C. Tonin, and A. D'Este. 1989. Locomotor strategies preceding independent walking: Prospective study of neurological and language development in 424 cases. *Developmental Medicine and Child Neurology* 31(1):25–34.

Bower, E., and D. McLellan. 1992. Effect of increased exposure to physiotherapy on skill acquisition of children with cerebral palsy. *Developmental Medicine and Child Neurology* 34(1):25–39.

Brann, A. 1988. The effects of acute total and prolonged partial asphyxia on the central nervous system of the fetus, neonate and juvenile rhesus monkey. In *Perinatal asphyxia, its role in developmental deficits in children*. Proceedings of a symposium held at Toronto, Ontario, October 26, 1988. American Academy for Cerebral Palsy and Developmental Medicine.

Brooks, S. 1990. Hip joint limitation: Contribution to sacral sitting. *Developmental Medicine and Child Neurology* October:43.

Brooks, S. 1994. Suggestions from the field: Hip joint limitation contribution to sacral sitting. *Pediatric Physical Therapy* (Winter):92.

Cailliet, R. 1966. *Shoulder pain*. Philadelphia: F. A. Davis.

Cornwall, M. 1984. Biomechanics of noncontractile tissue: A review. *Physical Therapy* 64(12): 1869–73.

Costello, A., P. Hamilton, J. Baudin, J. Townsend, B. Bradford, A. Stewart, and E. Reynolds. 1988. Prediction of neurodevelopmental impairment at four years from brain ultrasound appearance of very preterm infants. *Developmental Medicine and Child Neurology* 30:711–22.

Cusick, B. 1990. Progressive casting and splinting for lower extremity deformities in children with neuromotor dysfunction. Tucson, AZ: *Therapy Skill Builders*.

Cyriax, J. 1982. *Textbook of orthopedic medicine: Diagnosis of soft tissue lesions.* Vol. 1, 8th ed. London: Bailliere-Tindall.

Damiano, D., L. Kelly, and C. Vaughn. 1996. Effects of quadriceps femoris muscle strengthening on crouch gait in children with spastic diplegia. *Physical Therapy* 75(8):100–23.

Daniels, L., and C. Worthingham. 1972. *Muscle testing.* Philadelphia: W. B. Saunders.

Davis, J., and D. Kalousek. 1988. Fetal akinesia deformation sequence in previable fetuses. *American Journal Medical Genetics* 29(1):77–87.

Demilio, P. 1983. Periventricular-intraventricular hemorrhage in the neonate: A review. *Physical Therapy and Occupational Therapy in Pediatrics* 3:45–56.

DiFabio, R. 1992. Efficacy of manual therapy. *Physical Therapy* 72(12):853–64.

DiFabio, R. P. 1986. Clinical assessment of manipulation and mobilization of the spine: A critical review of the literature. *Physical Therapy* 66:55–63.

Doody, S., and J. Waterland. 1970. Shoulder movements during abduction in the scapular plane. *Archives of Physical Medicine Rehabilitation* 51:595.

Dunbar, D., F. Horak, J. Macpherson, and D. Rushmer. 1986. Neural control of quadripedal and bipedal stance: Implications for the evolution of erect posture. *American Journal of Physical Anthropology* 69(1):93–105.

Elveru, R., J. Rothstein, and R. Lamb. 1988. Goniometric reliability in a clinical setting; subtalor and ankle joint measurements. *Physical Therapy* 88:672–77.

Ely, L. W., and M. C. Mensor. 1962. Studies on the immobilization of the normal joints. *Surgery in Gynecology and Obstetrics* 57:212–15.

Engel, G., and L. Staheli. 1974. The natural history of torsion and other factors influencing gait in childhood: A study of the angle of gait, tibial torsion, knee, ankle hip rotation, and development of the arch in normal children. *Clinical Orthopedics and Related Research* 99:12–17.

Enneking, W., and M. Horowitz. 1972. The intra-articular effects of immobilization on the human knee. *Journal of Bone and Joint Surgery* 54a:973–85.

Esch, D., and M. Lepley. 1971. *Evaluation of joint motion: Methods of measurement and recording.* Minneapolis: University of Minnesota Press.

Evans, E. B., G. W. Eggers, J. K. Butler, and J. Blumel. 1960. Experimental immobilization of rat knee joints. *Journal of Bone and Joint Surgery* 42a:737–58.

Fabry, G., G. McEwen, and A. Shands. 1973. Torsion of the femur. *Journal of Bone and Joint Surgery* 55A(8):1725–38.

Folio, M., and R. Fewel. 1983. *Developmental motor scales*. Allen, TX: DLM Teaching Resources.

Frankenburg, W., and J. Dodds. 1967. The Denver developmental screening test. *Journal of Pediatrics* 71:181.

Frankel, V. H., and M. Nordin. 1980. *Basic biomechanics of the skeletal system*. Philadelphia: Lea and Febiger.

Frankel, V. H. 1973. Biomechanics of the knee. In *The Knee Joint*, edited by O. Ingiverson, New York: Elsevier.

Frankel, V. H., A. H. Burstein, and D. B. Brooks. 1971. Biomechanics of internal derangement of the knee: Pathomechanics as determined by analysis of the instant centers of motion. *Journal of Bone and Joint Surgery* 53a:945–62.

Freedman, L., and R. Munroe. 1966. Abduction of the arm in the scapular plane: Scapular and glenohumeral movements. *Journal of Bone and Joint Surgery* 48a(8):150.

Gate, V., M. Stefanova-Uzunova, L. Stamatova, and I. Ivonov. 1986. Excitation-contraction latency in the muscles of children and adults. *Developmental Medicine and Child Neurology* 28:642–5.

Gesell, A., and C. Amatruda. 1947. *Developmental diagnosis*. New York: Hoeber.

Giannestras, N. 1973. *Foot disorders: medical and surgical management*. Philadelphia: Lea and Febiger.

Guiliani, C. 1991. *Theories of motor control: New concepts for physical therapy. Contemporary management of motor control problems*. Alexandria, VA: Foundation of Physical Therapy.

Haas, S., C. Epps, and J. Adams. 1973. Normal ranges of hip motion in the newborn. *Clinical Orthopedics and Related Research* 91:114–18.

Hadders-Algra, M., B. Tuwen, and H. Hursjes. 1986. Neurologically deviant newborns: Neurological and behavioural development at the age of six years. *Developmental Medicine and Child Neurology* 28:569–78.

Hadler, N., P. Curtis, D. Gillings, and S. Stinnett. 1987. A benefit of spinal manipulation as adjunctive therapy for acute low back pain: A stratified controlled trail. *Spine* 12(7):702–6.

Harris, S., and B. Lundgren. 1991. Joint mobilization for children with central nervous system disorders: Indications and precautions. *Physical Therapy* 71(12):890–96.

Hensinger, R., and E. Jone. 1982. Developmental orthopedics I: The lower limb. *Developmental Medicine and Child Neurology* 24:95–116.

Hoesli, B. 1988. Effects of mobilization on hip flexion range in a child with cerebral palsy. Unpublished Senior Paper, St. Louis University. Presented at the APTA National Conference, 1989.

Hoffer, M. 1980. Joint motion limitation in newborns. *Clinical Orthopedics and Related Research* 148:94–6.

Holland, T. 1985. Coupling Pnf and joint mobilization. In *Proprioceptive neuromuscular facilitation*, edited by D. Holland, M. Ionta, and B. Myers. 3d ed. Philadelphia: Harper & Row.

Johnson, A., and H. Ashurst. 1989. Is popliteal angle measurement useful in early identification of cerebral palsy? *Developmental Medicine and Child Neurology* 31(4):457–65.

Johnston, R. C., and G. L. Smidt. 1970. Hip motion measurements for selected activities of daily living. *Clinical Orthopedics* 72:205.

Jordan, R., J. Cusack, and B. Resseque. 1983. *Foot function and its relationship to posture in pediatric patients with cerebral palsy and other neuromotor disorders.* Lecture notes from Langer Biomechanics Group, Inc.

Kaltenborn, F. 1976. *Manual therapy of the extremity joints.* Oslo, Norway: Olaf Norlis Bokhandel.

Kandell, E., and J. Schwartz. 1984. *Principles of neural science.* New York: Elsevier/North Holland.

Kapandji, I. A. 1970. *The physiology of the joints.* Volume 2. Baltimore: Williams & Wilkins.

Kendall, F., and E. McCreary. 1983. *Muscles testing and function.* 3d ed. Baltimore: Williams & Wilkins.

Kessler, R., and D. Hertling. 1983. *Management of common musculoskeletal disorders.* Philadelphia: Harper & Row.

Knutsson, E. 1980. Restraint of spastic muscles in different types of movement. In *Spasticity: Disordered motor control*, edited by R. Feldman, R. Young and W. Koella. Chicago: Year Book Medical Publishers.

Kottke, F. 1966. The effects of limitation of activity upon the human body. *Journal of American Medical Association* 196:825–30.

Kramer, J., and A. MacPhail. 1994. Relationships among measures of walking efficiency, gross motor ability, and isokinetic strength in adolescents with cerebral palsy. *Pediatric Physical Therapy* Spring 6(1):3–9.

Lacey, J., D. Henderson-Smart, and D. Edwards. 1990. A longitudinal study of early leg postures in preterm infants. *Developmental Medicine and Child Neurology* 32(2):151–63.

Lacey, J., D. Henderson-Smart, D. Edwards, and B. Storey. 1985. Early development of head control in preterm infants. *Early Human Development* 51(3-4):199–212.

Lee, C. 1977. *Forces acting to derotate exaggerated femoral antetorsion in the newborn hip*. Thesis of Fellowship UCP Research: Ed. Foundation NY Childrens Hospital, Stanford, 1977.

Leveau, B., and D. Bernhardt. 1984. Developmental biomechanics: Effect of forces on the growth, development, and maintenance of the human body. *Physical Therapy* 64(12):1874–82.

Lien-Mueller, M. 1989. Effects of joint mobilization techniques on gait pattern and range of motion in three children with spastic hemiplegia. University of Wisconsin: Master's Thesis.

MacConnail, M., and J. Basmajian. 1969. *Muscles and movement: A basis for human kinesiology*. Baltimore: Williams & Wilkins.

Mackinnon, J. 1988. Osteoporosis: A review. *Physical Therapy* 68(10):1533.

Maitland, G. 1977. *Peripheral manipulation*. Vol. 2. Boston: Butterworths.

Malina, R. 1988. Racial/ethnic variation in the motor development and performances of American children. *Canadian Journal of Sport Science* 13(2):136–43.

Mattles, A. 1965. The newborn hip guide: Technique of localizing the head of the newborn femur on roentgenograms. *New York State Journal of Medicine* 65:2345–50.

Mayfield, J., R. Johnson, and R. Kilcoyne. 1976. The ligaments of the human wrist and their functional significance. *Anatomy Record* 186(3):417.

McClenaghan, B., L. Thombs, and M. Milner. 1992. Effects of seat surface inclination on postural stability and function of the upper extremities of children with cerebral palsy. *Developmental Medicine and Child Neurology* 34(1):40–8.

McCrea, J. 1985. *Pediatric orthopedics of the lower extremity: An instructional handbook*. Mount Kisco: Futura Publishing Co.

McEwan, M., F. Dihoff, and G. Brosvic. 1991. Early infant crawling experience is reflected in later motor skills development. *Perceptual Motor Skills* 72(1):75–9.

Milgrom, C., M. Giladi, A. Simkin, H. Stein, J. Kashtan, J. Margulies, R. Steinberg, and Z. Aharonson. 1985. The normal range of subtalor inversion and eversion in young males as measured by three different techniques. *Foot and Ankle* 6(3):143–45.

Milner-Brown, H. S., and R. D. Penn. 1979. Pathophysiological mechanisms in cerebral palsy *Journal of Neurology, Neurosurgery and Psychiatry* 42:606.

Moore, J. C. 1986. Neonatal neuropathology. *Physical and Occupational Therapy in Pediatrics* 6(3–4):55–90.

Moritz, V. 1979. Evaluation of manipulation and other manual therapy. *Scandinavian Journal of Rehabilitation Medicine* 11:173–79.

Nashner, L. M. 1976. Adapting reflexes controlling human posture. *Experimental Brain Research* 26:59.

Nashner, L. M.. 1977. Fixed patterns of rapid postural responses among leg muscles during stance. *Experimental Brain Research* 30:13.

Nashner, L. M. 1981. Analysis of stance posture in humans. In *Handbook of Behavioural Neurobiology*, edited by A. Towe and E. Luschei. New York: Plenum Press.

Nashner, L. M., A. Shumway-Cook, and O. Marin. 1983. Stance postural control in select groups of children with cerebral palsy, deficits in sensory organization and muscular coordination. *Experimental Brain Research* 49:393–409.

Nelson, K. 1988. Perspective on the role of perinatal asphyxia in neurologic outcome. In *Perinatal asphyxia: Its role in developmental deficits in children*. Proceedings of a Symposium held at Toronto, Ontario, October 26, 1988. American Academy for Cerebral Palsy and Developmental Medicine.

Nicholson, G. G. 1987. The effects of passive joint mobilization on pain and hypomobility associated with adhesive capsulitis of the shoulder. *The Journal of Orthopedic and Sports Physical Therapy* 4:238–46.

Norkin, C., and P. Levangie. 1983. *Joint structure and function*. Philadelphia: F. A. Davis.

Nwaobi, O. 1987. Seating orientations and upper extremity function in children with cerebral palsy. *Physical Therapy* Aug 67(8):1209–12.

Nwaobi, O., D. Hobson, and S. Taylor. 1969. Mechanical and anatomic hip flexion angles on seating children with cerebral palsy. *Archives of Physical Medicine Rehabilitation* 69(4):265–67.

Olson, V. L. 1987. Evaluation of joint mobilization treatment: A method. *Physical Therapy* 67:351–6.

Ottenbacher, K., and R. P. DiFabio. 1985. Efficacy of spinal manipulations/mobilization therapy: A meta-analysis. *Spine* 10:833–7.

Pape, K., and J. Wigglesworth. 1979. *Haemorrhage, ischaemia, and the perinatal brain.* London: Heinemann.

Perry, J., M. M. Hoffer, and P. Giovan. 1974. Gait analysis of the triceps surae in cerebral palsy: A preoperative and postoperative clinical and electromyographic study. *Journal of Bone and Joint Surgery* 56a:511.

Phelps, E., L. Smith, and A. Hallum. 1985. Normal ranges of hip motion of infants between nine and 24 months of age. *Developmental Medicine and Child Neurology* 27:785–92.

Pitkow, R. 1975. External rotation contracture of the extended hip. *Clinical Orthopedics and Related Research* 110:139–45.

Radin, E. L., S. R. Simon, R. M. Rose, and I. L. Paul. 1979. *Practical biomechanics for the orthopedic surgeon.* New York: John Wiley and Sons.

Rana, M. 1984. *Key facts in embryology.* New York: Churchill Livingstone.

Raney, R., and Brashear. 1971. *Shands's handbook of orthopaedic surgery.* 8th ed. St. Louis, MO: Mosby.

Rang, M., R. Silver, and J. De La Garza. 1986. *Cerebral palsy.* In *Pediatric orthopedics*, edited by W. Lovell. 2d ed. Philadelphia: Lippincott.

Robson, P. 1984. Prewalking locomotor movements and their use in predicting standing and walking. *Child Care Health and Development* 10(5):317–30.

Root, M., W. Orien, and J. Weed. 1977. *Normal and abnormal function of the foot: Clinical biomechanics.* Vol. 2. Los Angeles: Clinical Biomechanics Corporation.

Rose, S., and J. Rothstein. 1982. Muscle mutability—Part I: General concepts and adaptations to altered patterns of use. *Physical Therapy* 62(12):1773–87.

Rosenflack, A., and S. Andreasson. 1980. Impaired regulation of force and firing pattern of single motor units in patients with spasticity. *Journal of Neurology, Neurosurgery and Psychiatry* 43:907–16.

Rothstein, J., P. Miller, and R. Roettger. 1983. Goniometric reliability in a clinical setting: Elbow and knee measurements. *Physical Therapy* 63(10):1611–15.

Sadler, T. W. 1985. *Langman's Medical Embryology.* 5th ed. Baltimore: Williams & Wilkins.

Salter, R. 1978. *Textbook of disorders and injuries of the musculoskeletal system.* 2d ed. Baltimore: Williams & Wilkins.

Saltin, B., and S. Landen. 1975. Work capacity, muscle strength, and SDH activity in both legs of hemiparetic patients and patients with Parkinson's Disease. *Scandinavian Journal of Clinical Lab Investigations* 35:531–8.

Sarafian, S., J. Melsmed, and G. Goshgarian. 1977. Study of wrist motion in flexion and extension. *Clinical Orthopedics* 126:153.

Saunders, H. 1985. *Evaluation, treatment, and prevention of musculoskeletal disorders.* Minneapolis: Viking Press.

Sgarlato, T. 1971. *A compendium of biomechanics.* San Francisco: California College of Podiatric Medicine.

Singleton, M. C., and B. F. Leveau. 1975. The hip joint: Stability and stress: A review. *Physical Therapy* 55:9.

Slaten, D. 1981. Muscle fiber types and their development in the human fetus. *Physical & Occupational Therapy Pediatrics* 47(1).

Spielholz, N. 1982. Skeletal muscle: A review of its development in vivo and in vitro. *Physical Therapy* 62(12):1757–62.

Staheli, L. 1977. The prone hip extension test. *Clinical Orthopaedics and Related Research* 123:12–15.

Staudt, L., and W. Peacock. 1989. Selective posterior rhizotomy for treatment of spastic cerebral palsy. *Pediatric Physical Therapy* 1:1.

Steindler, A. 1973. *Kinesiology of the human body.* Springfield, IL: Charles C. Thomas.

Stewart, A., E. Reynolds, P. Hope, P. Hamilton, J. Randu, A. De La Castello, B. Bradford, and J. Wyatt. 1987. Probability of neurodevelopmental disorders estimated from ultrasound appearance of brains of very preterm infants. *Developmental Medicine and Child Neurology* 29:3–11.

Stokes, M., and A. Young. 1984. The contribution of reflex inhibition to arthrogenous muscle weakness. *Clinical Science* 67:7–14.

Stuberg, W., R. Fuchs, M. Wichita, J. Temme, and P. Kaplan. 1989. Comparison of femoral torsion assessment using goniometry and computerized tomography. *Pediatric Physical Therapy* Fall 1(3):115–20.

Stuberg, W., and W. Metcalf. 1988. Reliability of quantitative muscle testing in healthy children and in children with Duchenne muscular dystrophy using a hand-held dynamometer. *Physical Therapy* 68(6):977–82.

Super, C. 1976. Environmental effects on motor development: The case of "African Infant Precocity." *Developmental Medicine and Child Neurology* 18(5):561–7.

Sutherland, D., and L. Cooper. 1984. *Gait disorders in childhood and adolescence*. Baltimore: Williams & Wilkins.

Sutherland, D., L. Cooper, and D. Daniel. 1980. The role of the plantar flexors in normal walking. *Journal of Bone and Joint Surgery* 62a:3.

Tachdjian, M. 1971. *Pediatric Orthopedics*. Philadelphia: W. B. Saunders.

Tang, A., and W. Aymer. 1981. Abnormal force EMG relations in paretic limbs of hemiparetic human subjects. *Journal of Neurology, Neurosurgery and Psychiatry* 44:690–98.

Tardieu, G., and C. Tardieu. 1987. Cerebral palsy: Mechanical evaluation and conservative correction of limb joint contractures. *Clinical Orthopedics and Related Research* 219:63–70.

Tax, H. 1985. *Podopediatrics*, 2d ed. Baltimore: Williams & Wilkins.

Thelen, E., D. Corbetta, K. Kamm, J. Spencer, K. Schneider, and R. Zernicke. 1993. The transition to reaching: Mapping intention and intrinsic dynamics. *Child Development* 64(4):1058–98.

Thornton, K. 1992. Screening Moroccan infants using the Wolanski Gross Motor Evaluation: A pilot study. *Studies In Human Ecology* 10:121–6.

Threlkeld, A. 1992. The effects of manual therapy on connective tissue. *Physical Therapy* 72(12):893–902.

Van Sant, A. F. 1989. The child with orthopaedic problems. In *Manual of Physical Therapy*, by O. Payton. New York: Churchill Livingstone.

Van Sant, A. F. 1988. Age differences in movement patterns used by children to rise from a supine position to erect stance. *Physical Therapy* 68(9): 1330–7.

Vaughan, V. 1989. Effects of upper limb immobilization on isometric muscle strength, movement time, and triphasic electromyographic characteristics. *Physical Therapy* 69(2):119–29.

Viljoen, D., G. Versfeld, and P. Beighton. 1989. Osteogenesis imperfecta with congenital joint contractures. *Clinical Genetics* 36(2): 122–6.

Volpe, J. 1988. Pathophysiology of perinatal hypoxic/ischemic brain injury. In *Perinatal asphyxia: Its role in developmental deficits in children*. Proceedings of a Symposium held at Toronto, Ontario, October 26, 1988. American Academy for Cerebral Palsy and Developmental Medicine.

Wisman, J., F. Veldpaus, and J. Janssen. 1980. A three dimensional mathematical model of the knee joint. *Journal of Biomechanics* 13:677.

Woo, S. L., J. V. Mathews, and W. H. Akeson. 1975. Connective tissue response to immobility. *Arthritis Rheumatology* 18(3):257–64.

Youm, Y. 1978. Kinematics of the wrist: An experimental study of radial-ulnar deviation and flexion-extension. *Journal of Bone and Joint Surgery* 6a(4):423.

Youm, Y. 1979. Biomechanical analysis of forearm pronation-supination and elbow flexion-extension. *Journal of Biomechanics* 12:245.

Math
Fundamentals
A Review
Fourth Edition

Ellen Freedman
Kelly A. Jackson
Virginia Licata
Barbara Jane Sparks
Camden County College

McGraw-Hill **Custom Publishing**

New York St. Louis San Francisco Auckland Bogotá
Caracas Lisbon London Madrid Mexico Milan Montreal
New Delhi Paris San Juan Singapore Sydney Tokyo Toronto

Math Fundamentals, Fourth Edition
A Review

McGraw-Hill's Primis Custom Series consists of products that are produced from camera-ready copy. Peer review, class testing, and accuracy are primarily the responsibility of the author(s).

7 8 9 0 QPD QPD 0 9 8

ISBN-13: 978-0-07-304725-6
ISBN-10: 0-07-304725-2

Editor: Robin E. Havens
Production Editor: Kathy Phelan
Printer/Binder: Quebecor World